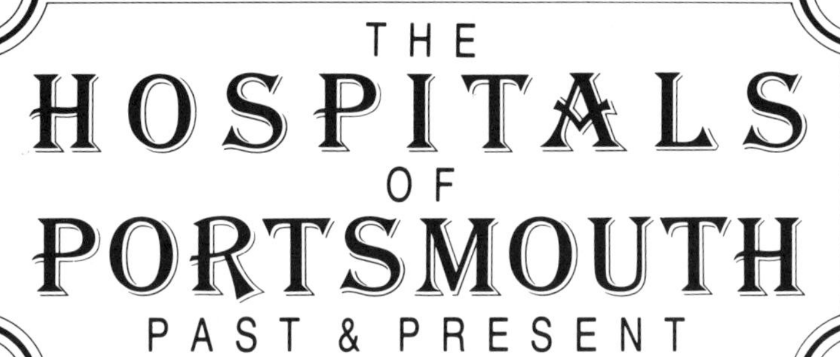

THE HOSPITALS OF PORTSMOUTH PAST & PRESENT

BY MOLLY GANGE

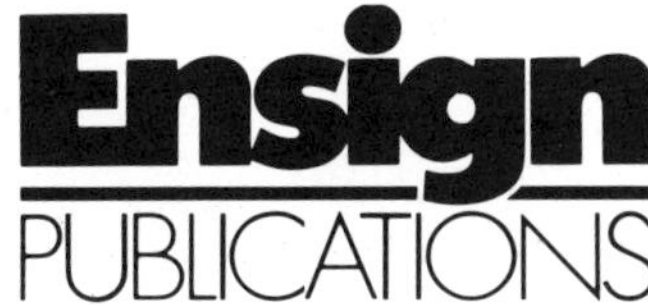
Ensign PUBLICATIONS

Published by Ensign Publications
2 Redcar Street, Shirley Precinct
Southampton SO1 5LL

First published 1988

ISBN 1-85455-001-2

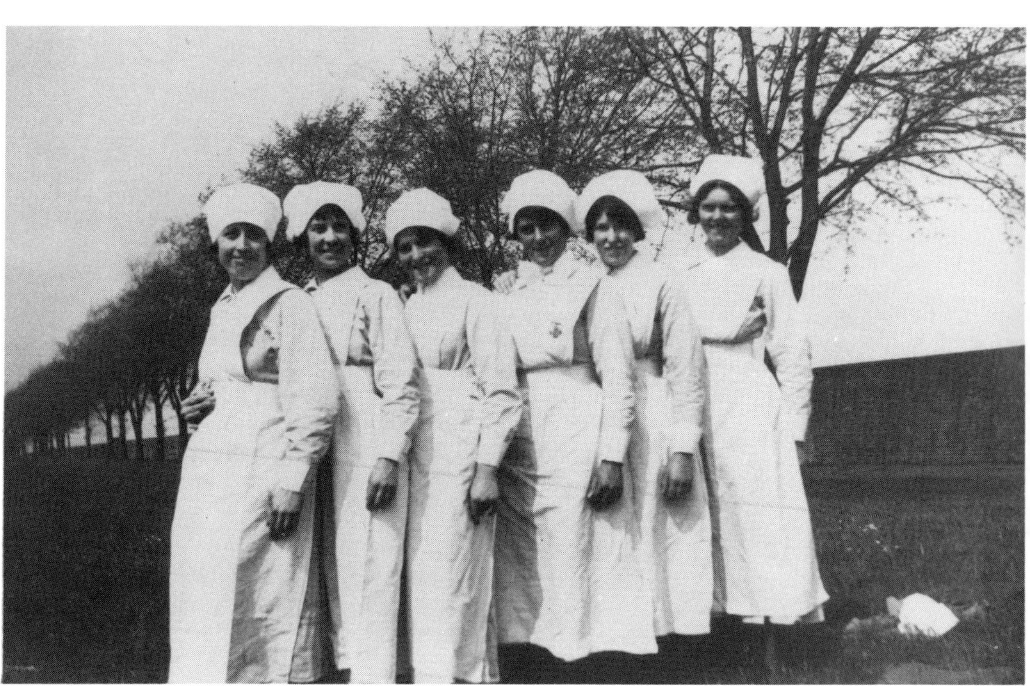

The first Hospital in Portsmouth was the Hospital of St Nicholas, or as it was better known at that time, the Domus Dei. Founded by Peter de Rupibus, Bishop of Winchester it gave sanctuary to the earliest known patients and the poor from 1212 till 1540. First there were twelve brothers, then six brothers and six sisters who were responsible for the nursing. The arrangement of the beds across each side of a central corridor seemed to be similar to that of the older hospitals today.

Another similarity was the constant need for funds. One of the difficulties the brothers had to surmount was competition from the church of St Thomas founded five years before. The Domus Dei was popular with the people and the church soom found their income from the offerings received from their congregation was reduced. So something had to be done. The two establishments entered into an arrangement to equalise their incomes.

The Domus Dei had to pay the church £1 per annum and agree not to hold services on Sundays and the eight Saints Days. When services were attended by the general public all offerings had to be handed over. Also, and this does sound strange but no doubt had significance at the time, they had to agree to have a lighter bell and only ring it on special occasions.

In spite of all these restrictions sufficient funds were raised for the care of the sick to continue until the dissolution of the monasteries by Henry VIII in 1540.

The building then fell into disrepair and was used as a store until it was later restored and became Government House. It was put to this use until early in the nineteenth century. The last Governor of Portsmouth was the Duke of Connaught who bridged the years when he laid the foundation stone of the enlarged Royal Hospital in 1899. One of the wards was named after him so the connection with the Demus Dei remained until the Royal was demolished in 1984.

The Domus Dei building was badly damaged by fire bombs in 1941 but has now been restored. One of the windows depicts Peter de Rupibus, so the memory of the original hospital has been kept alive. On Governors Green near the Clarence Pier stands a lasting monument to the care of the sick in Portsea throughout the centuries.

The Domus Dei was not the only hospital in Portsea in these days. Little is known of the others but one was called the Chapel of our Lady of Close. It is thought that the sick were cared for there and it is reputed to have stood on the land later occupied by the Coleworth Barracks; that is west of St Georges' Road where it joins Warblington Road. Also on that site in 1679 stood the first military hospital in the country. It was not there very long as the buildings were incorporated into the Coleworth Barracks which opened in 1694. So with a life of only fifteen years it must have been one of the shortest-lived hospitals in Portsmouth.

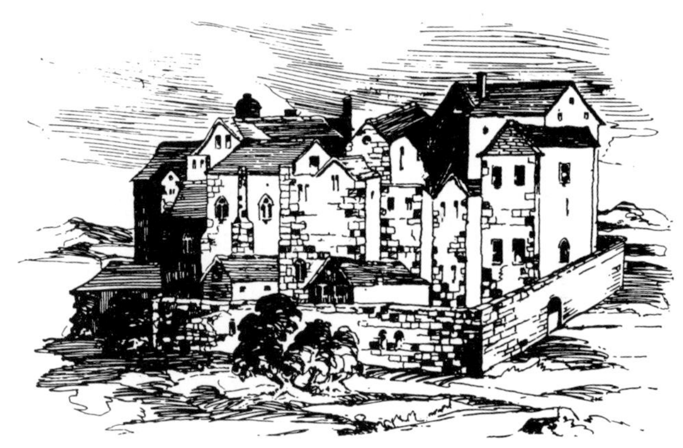

The Domus Dei.

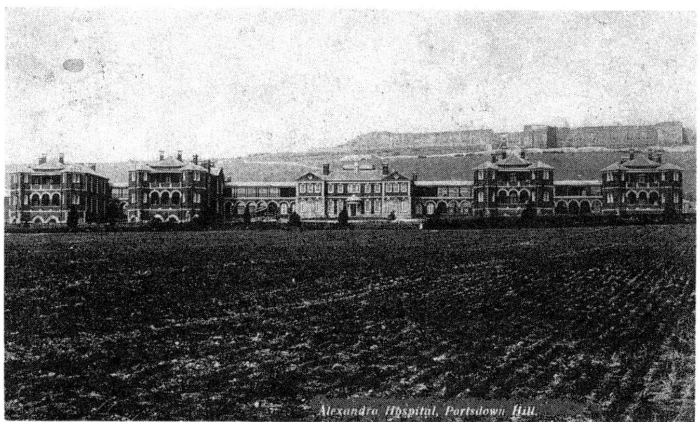

The first Military Hospital.

There were other military hospitals after this one. They do not seem to be well documentated but it is possible to see them marked on old maps of the area. One which does not seem to be on any map but which is often mentioned in accounts of that time was a military hospital at Cambridge Junction. It may have been of short duration or too small to be included.

The hospital near H.M.S. Nelson between Anglesey Road and Mill Dam Road near Lion Place is clearly marked on the map dated 1860 and was a good size. It is dated 1853 and described as a garrison hospital. It was reputed to have had accommodation for three hundred patients.

Also on the same map is the Royal Marine Infirmary. There is no date here but it is in the area covered by H.M.S. Vernon and was near the Gunwarf Barracks facing Gunwarf Road.

On the Survey map of 1876/77 there was a military families hospital at Hilsea. This was attached to the Hilsea Artillery Barracks and was still in use well into this century.

The services had a maternity home in Portsmouth. "Bowlands" will bring back memories to many and it too lasted well into this century.

From 1745 the Navy was catered for at Gosport which explains the lack of hospitals for the senior service in Portsmouth. Although this is outside the area covered by this story its beginning is worth a mention.

From 1713 there was a Fortunes Hospital which was built on the site later occupied by Forton Barracks. This institution was owned by Nathaniel Jackson who contracted the "Commissioners for the Sick and Hurts" to treat patients for a fixed price per head. The system broke down because of 'gross irregularities', probably of a financial nature. So the R.N. Hospital at Haslar was built, initially designed to accommodate well over a thousand patients.

Another early hospital was outside the city walls. It may have been on the site occupied by the Guildhall today, or where the Portsmouth Registrar's Office stands in St Michaels Road. Yet another position favoured by some researchers is near St Mary's Church. In any case it was outside the walls as lepers found sanctuary there. Apart from its name, the Chapel of St Mary Magdalene little is known about it.

During the war with France there was large wooden barracks near Lion Terrace, Portsea. The Coleworth Barracks situation was reversed when they were demolished to make way for a military hospital in 1853. Their function changed again when the buildings were taken over by the Admiralty for the housing of personnel. Queen Alexandra Hospital on Portsdown Hill was then built to take its place.

Apart from the Military Hospitals there seems to have been a long gap when the only means of caring for the sick in Portsmouth was in their own homes. There were dispensaries; the best known in Portsea was the Portsmouth and Portsea Dispensary in St Georges Square which was opened in 1823. So it was not until the Royal Portsmouth Portsea and Gosport Hospital was opened in 1849 that in-patient care became possible.

With the opening of the Royal there seemed to be a general increase in awareness of the needs of the poor and the sick. The next hospital to be opened was St James Hospital, Milton. At that time it was called the Borough of Portsmouth Lunatic Asylum and was originally intended to house four hundred and ten patients. It was three years in the building and was opened in 1879.

In 1882 the Milton Hospital for the treatment of infectious diseases was opened. Initially it consisted of out-patients, one administration block and two pavilions in which twenty-four patients would be nursed. No smallpox patients were admitted as these were cared for in a Humphrey's Iron Building. This was the Locks Hospital for Smallpox and was under the direction of Dr A. Mearns Frazer, and situated from 1900 to 1911 on ground later occupied by Langstone Hospital for the treatment of tuberculosis. By 1911 the incidence of smallpox was greatly reduced because of the increased use of vaccination.

Two years later the Eye and Ear Hospital was founded. Initially it was quite small, use having been made of an already existing house. The staff consisted of one nurse. It was situated near the old King Williams Gate which stood between the Common and Old Portsmouth, around the area now occupied by Pembroke Gardens. So in 1884 another hospital came into being.

Still in the nineteenth century came St Mary's founded in 1898 whilst Queen Alexandra Hospital, opened in 1908 takes us into the twentieth century.

In 1911 the Langstone Hospital for the treatment of early cases of tuberculosis was opened. Like the Locks Hospital which preceded it it was under the direction of Dr A. Mearns Frazer M.D. It had six beds, three for men and three for women in the first instance.

In 1920 the Municipal Maternity Hospital opended. On the corner of Elm Grove and Victoria Road South there was accommodation for fourteen patients. Dr R.K. Ford was superintendent with Miss Cranford as Matron. The building was originally a private house and was considered to be particularly suited for its use on more than one count. Apart from its size it was considered to be perfectly situated, in a central position with the tram cars passing the door. It was first acquired on a lease but in 1921 was brought by the Corporation for £3,800.

It was described as a laying-in hospital for the reception of mothers whose home circumstances were so poor that they could not be cared for there. Anyone enjoying an income of more than 60 shillings per week would not be admitted. The hospital was also a training school for four pupil midwives.

The hospital remained in Elm Grove for seven years, when it was transferred to Trafalgar Place, a turning off Clive Road behind Fratton Road. The Child Welfare Clinic was already there and the hospital was joined on to the clinic. It remained there until 1938 when it was closed down. The whole building was then taken over by the welfare department.

The next smaller hospital, the Eye and Ear, or to give it its correct title the Portsmouth and South Hants Eye and Ear Infirmary, was opened in 1884. It was preceded by the South Hants Dispensary for diseases of the Eye and Ear which had been opened in 1824. Like the General Dispensary which had been opened in 1823 it was situated in St Georges Square. So there may have been some connection between them; some historians believe they were joined.

The hospital began with one small house on the corner of a terrace of eight houses in Clarence View, Portsmouth. It had five rooms of which three were bedrooms. The staff consisted of two medical officers, Dr J. Ward Cousins and Dr Vernon Ford, and one nurse.

When the hospital was first considered there was a great deal of opposition to the project. The need for such a facility was in no doubt but the advisability of having another voluntary hospital in the area was. As in the days of the Domus Dei and St Thomas' Church, the idea of two institutions relying on the same people for funds was thought to be unwise. It was decided that the Royal Hospital could only lose by the arrangement, but facts proved otherwise. The first year saw the Eye and Ear with an income of £200, a third coming from the patients and the rest raised from the general public. At the same time the financial position of the Royal thrived.

The need for the service reflected in the account of the attendances. In the first year sixteen hundred individual patients were recorded and the attendances amounted to sixteen thousand. The main problem was a shortage of space. The income was improving but not enough to fund the extensive alterations needed. Patients waiting for treatment were standing in corridors, on the stairs and even outside in the rain. The estimated cost for each patient was only 2s2½d (about 11p) but still finances were over stretched.

The area of intake was wide — Petersfield, Bognor, Shedfield and Wickham but these outside districts donated very little to the running costs. The local people held fund raising events in the way of whist drives, concerts and no doubt bazaars to involve as many as possible. They were given wholehearted support in trying to keep the hospital going. As this was such a one sided affair it was decided in 1891 to ask each patient for a small payment towards their treatment.

The year before had seen some financial improvement as a visitor to Southsea gave £1,000 on the understanding that the out-patient accommodation would be improved. Could she have had some eye trouble during her holiday and perhaps was one of the unfortunates who had to wait in the rain?

Other voices were added to the pleas for support. Dr. Arthur Conan Doyle who was at that time a practitioner in Portsmouth added his voice to encourage the fund raising efforts whilst the press were using their influence to try to make the town aware of the hospital's need.

By 1892 the new out-patients department was opened at a cost of £1,300. The patients who now had no longer to wait in the rain or up the stairs had much to thank the anonymous lady for. In fact this was not the only time her generosity helped the hospital. The next year she agreed to once more give a donation. This time it was for beds, linen and furniture. She also financed some very necessary repairs to the building.

This benefactor was a shadowy figure and it is not known why her

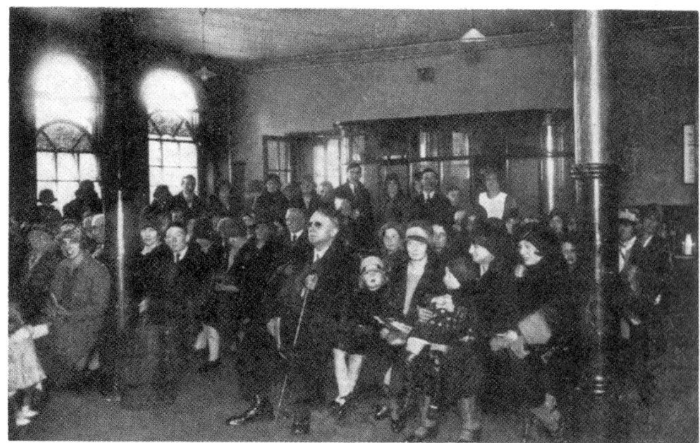

Waiting room. Eye and Ear Hospital 1920/22.

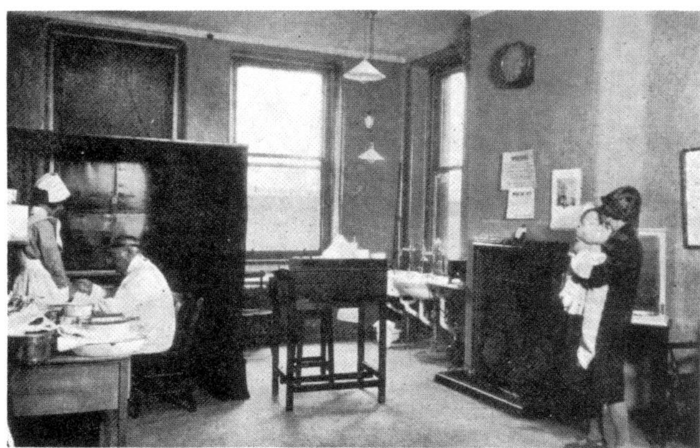

Eye and Ear out-patients Dept. 1920/30.

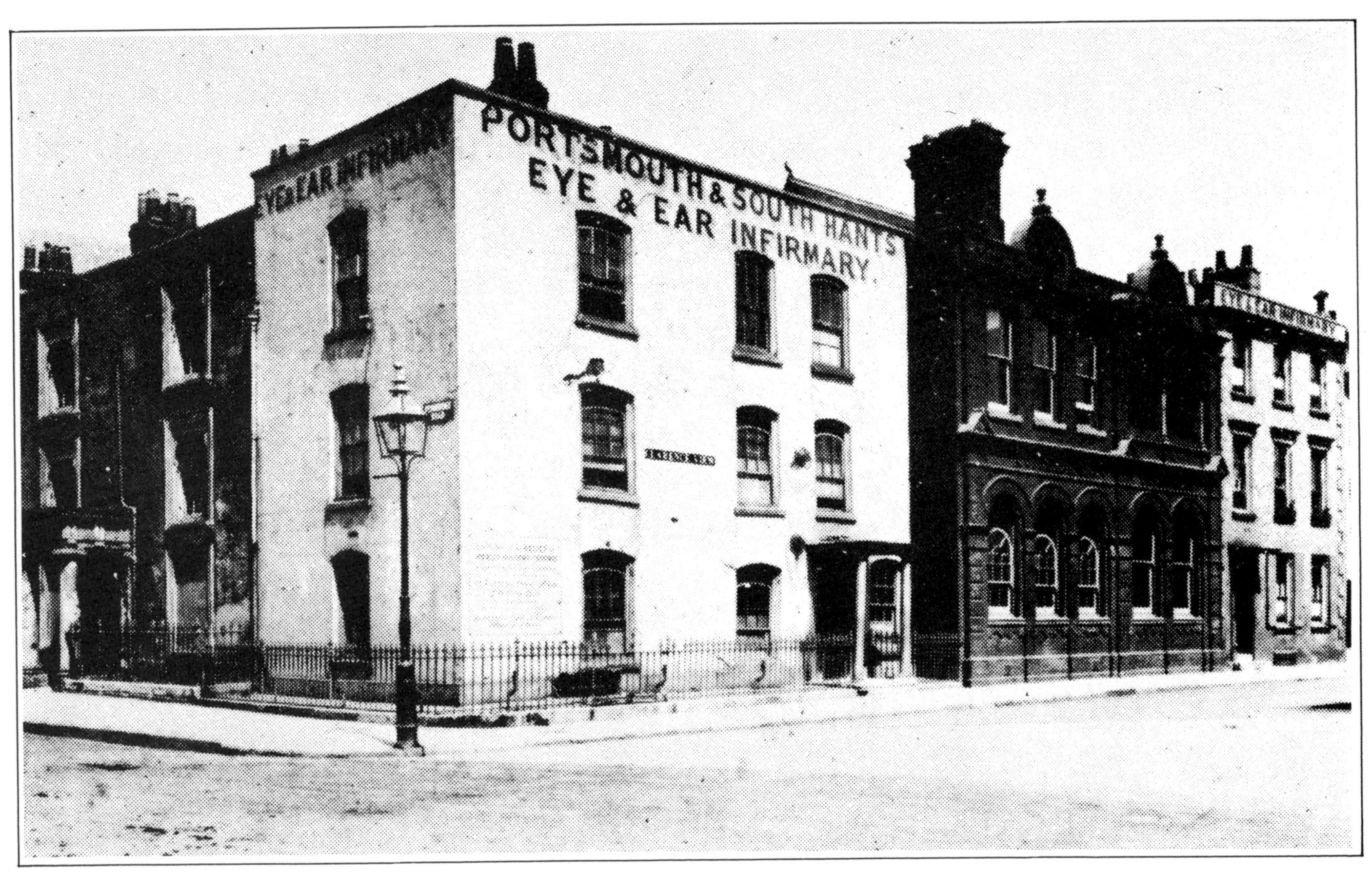

Eye and Ear Hospital 1898.

£1500 £1500
WANTED WANTED
TO COMPLETE
THE EXTENSION TO
THIS THIS
HOSPITAL HOSPITAL
Pembroke Road, Portsmouth.
6652.

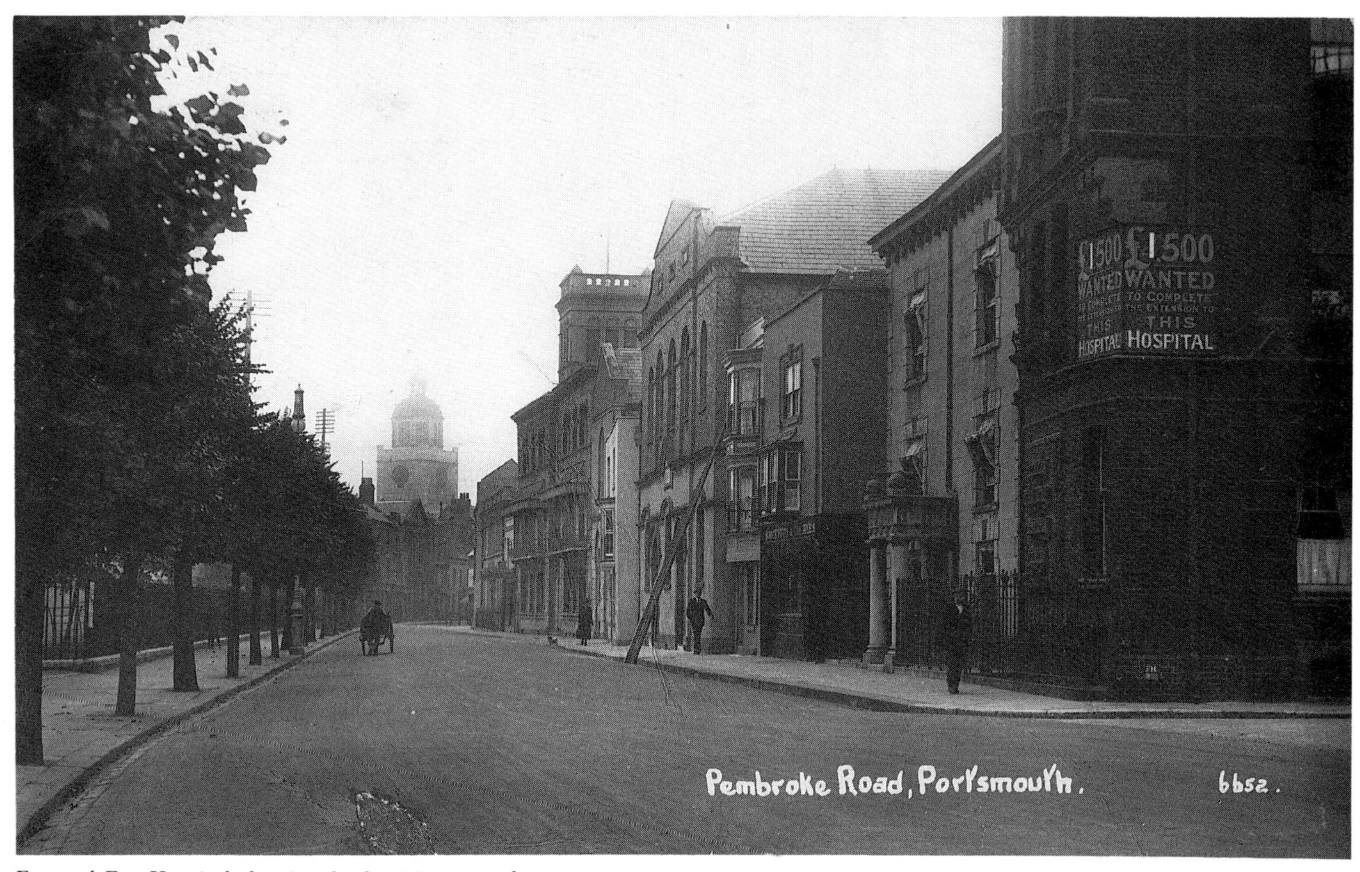

Eye and Ear Hospital showing fund raising appeal.

interest was aroused in the first place. Although she did not live locally she obviously had a genuine and practical interest in the welfare of the Eye and Ear.

As the popularity of the hospital grew it became obvious that further accommodation was now essential. The Committee had been gradually buying the rest of the houses in Clarence View Terrace and in 1910 they purchased the last one. But as usual the financial position was so precarious that acquiring the property depended on a fund raising event.

This was a Floral Fete which was held over a period of three days and raised over £1,000. This amount, when added to several legacies made it possible to start building.

In 1913 the foundation stone was laid by the chairman of the committee Mr Henry Dummer. The plans for the new wards were drawn up by a firm of Bloomsbury architects, Young and Hall; the estimated cost was £6,665. When the building was completed the institution was the largest of its kind south of Birmingham specialising in diseases of the eye and ear. It was decided its present title was no longer appropriate so it was renamed the Portsmouth and Southern Counties Eye and Ear Hospital, and this was the title given by H.R.H. Princess Henry of Battenburg when she opened the new building on July 22nd 1914.

The new building was geared to match the old one to which it was connected by a corridor. It was faced with red brick and the authorities were delighted with the result. In the basement there were four large stores and a small lift connecting them to the upper floors. On the ground floor was a consulting room, board room, kitchen, dispensary and nurses common room. The first and second floors both contain one large ward of eight beds, one of four beds and two single bedded wards. Mr Edwin Stevens left a legacy of £2,000 and as a memorial to him one of the wards was named Steven Ward.

With these two buildings there were now forty-eight beds in all. But these did not last long as far as the people of Portsmouth were

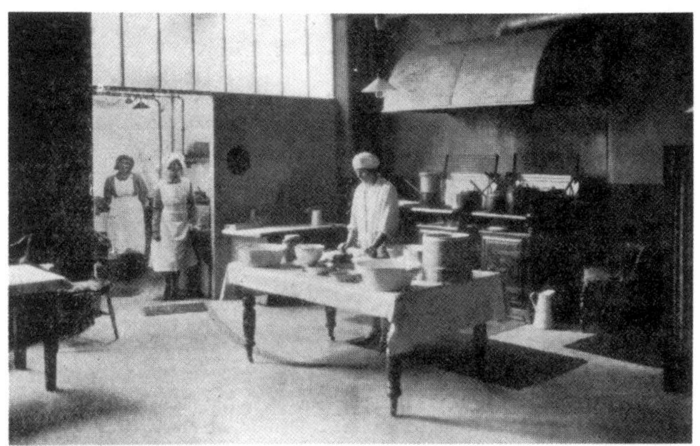

The Kitchens.

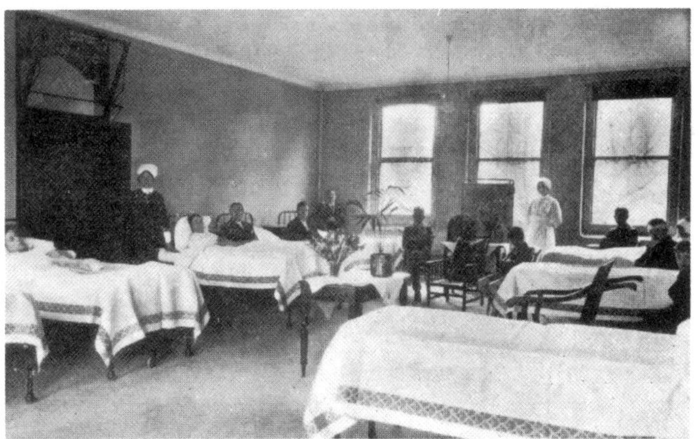

Mens Ward.

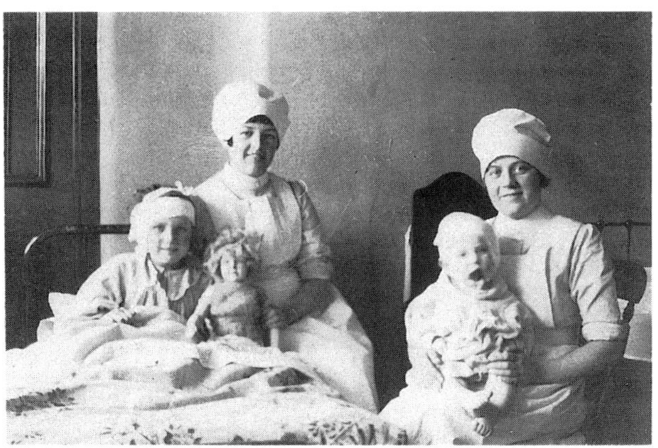

Small children recovering from Mastoid operation.

concerned. On the following October half the wards were taken over by the armed forces. This state of affairs considerably helped the financial position as they were paid for by the Ministry involved. To this was added the money from the Rose Flag Day, several legacies and contributions from the Hospital Saturday and Sunday Fund. By the end of the war for the first time the financial state was described as very satisfactory.

By this time it had become imperative that far more be spent on medical and surgical appliances. The nursing staff was also considerably under strength. Previously all tonsil and adenoid patients had been sent home on the day of their operation, a far from ideal arrangement. Mr Scott Ridout advocated a stay of twenty-four hours in summer and forty-eight in winter. Unfortunately this state of affairs was still continuing in 1932. Lack of beds and nurses were the problem.

Soon after the war the Royal Hospital suggested that both hospitals should come together under one management. If they did amalgamate it would have been necessary to considerably enlarge the Eye and Ear. On the other hand if the Royal tried to take in the Eye and Ear patients they would have little to offer in the way of facilities. In fact there seemed to be little of advantage and quite a lot to lose. So the idea was rejected. The matter was brought up again in 1929 but the answer was the same. Five years later they arrived at a compromise and each had a representative on their separate committees.

It was at one of these meetings that two interesting facts arose. Mr Scott Ridout had noticed that whenever there was an influx of appendicitis cases at the Royal the Eye and Ear had a similar increase in patients suffering from Mastoids. No reason was ever found for this any more than why Portsmouth had such a high number of cases with disease of the ear in general.

The hospital had a singularly unusual problem because of its nearness to the military barracks. The hospital was just outside the

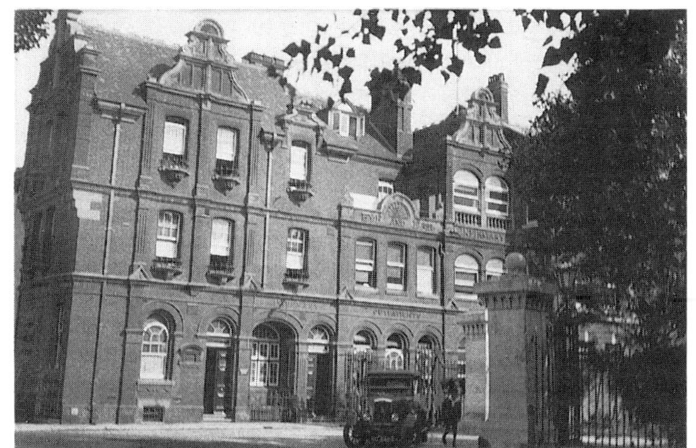

The hospital gates.

barracks and there was a dividing wall separating the garden from the barracks square. The two main gates were very close together and this often was too much for the soliders returning after a night out. They climbed the wrong one and were quite unable to work out why they were cut off from their goal. The nurses rounded them up and sat them in out-patients to await the arrival of the Military Police who escorted them back to their quarters. This was not an infrequent occurance but every time it happened they showed considerable surprise. As Staff Nurse Bailey said: "I couldn't open the gate and let them out. They were in such a state it was a wonder they got over safely in the first place."

Explaining why the out-patients clinics over-ran, Mr C.A. Scott Ridout the E.N.T. surgeon said that the lists were so variable, it was impossible to give appointments without considerably increasing the waiting list. Sometimes there were between eighty and one hundred patients at a session. Those who travelled long distances and had trains or boats to catch were seen first and this was far from popular with the local patients. The doctor never knew how many would attend and often worked from two o'clock until nine or ten at night. As this was after a morning spent in the theatre or on the wards, it made a very long day.

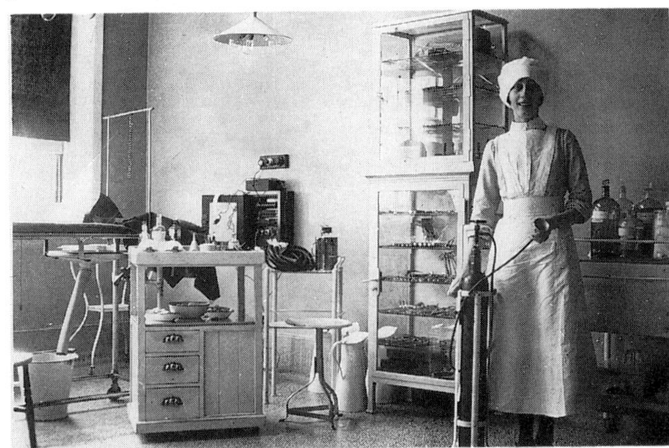

Treatment room out-patients dept.

Mr W.S. Inman, the eye surgeon made it clear that to run the clinic like a machine was not the answer. Time and sympathy was essential especially with children. This was demonstrated by the case of one patient. She realised this when recalling the care she received when as an eight year old she had a serious accident which left her nearly blind. After many visits during which she learnt to look on everyone as her friend she saw something bright in the doctors pocket. She asked what it was and when she was told to take it out she did so. At the time she thought how silly to make such a fuss about a small thing like that, everyone was so delighted. It was some years later when she realised how near she was to being blind for the rest of her life. From that time her sight improved and she was able to train as a nurse herself.

In 1930 a special appeal was launched and a booklet was printed with a very detailed account of the finances over the past forty-six years. They also listed the patients treated. From 1884-1930 there were 18,396 in-patients, 136,689 out-patients and 43,008 operations. Income — ordinary income = £68,984 — legacies £20,373 15s 1d. The habit of giving vast sums of money to the last penny gave the impression, no doubt correctly, of very careful housekeeping.

At the same time they gave a full shopping list which they hoped to achieve by the appeal. It consisted of The conversion of the previously bought "Trafalgar House" into the new nurses home, the installation of a patients lift and outside fire escape, building equipment and sterilising room, the provision of a servants hall and the alterations to the old nurses home to provide three more wards.

Seven years later things were improving so much it was estimated that if regular contributions increased form 2d to 3d per week all would be well.

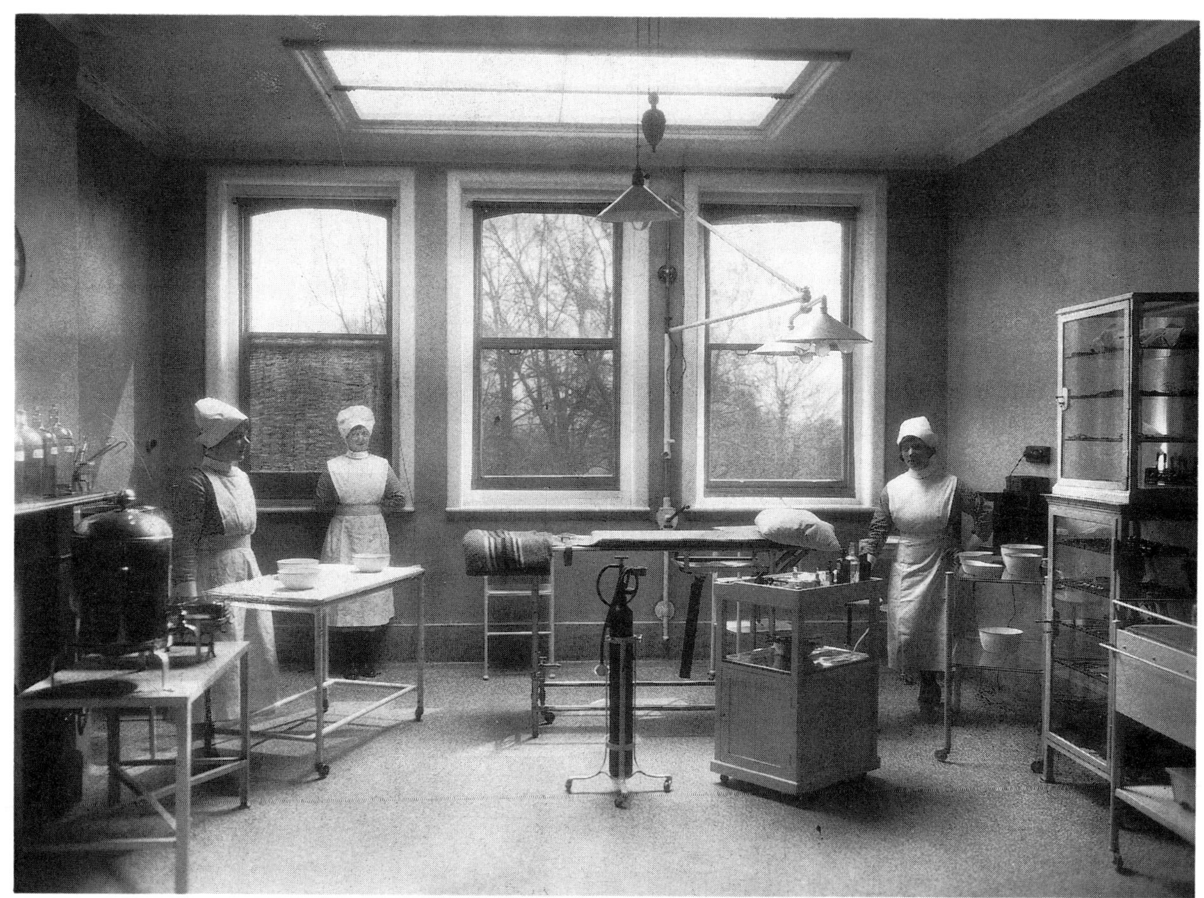

Operating Theatre 1923/24.

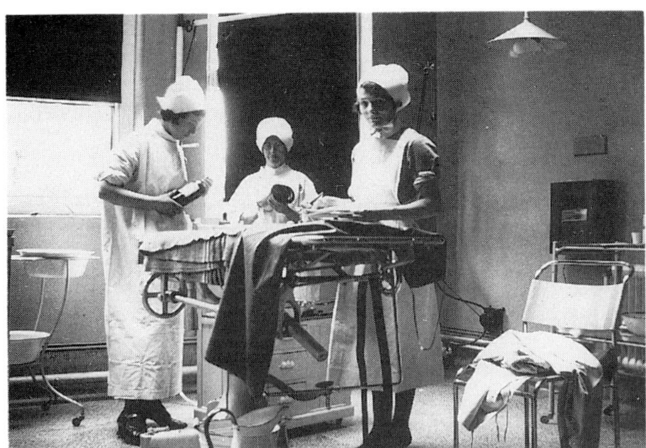

Preparing for a minor operation in out-patients dept.

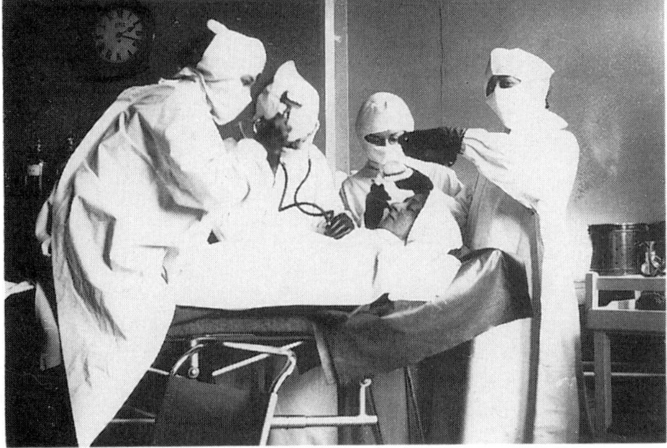

Operation in progress.

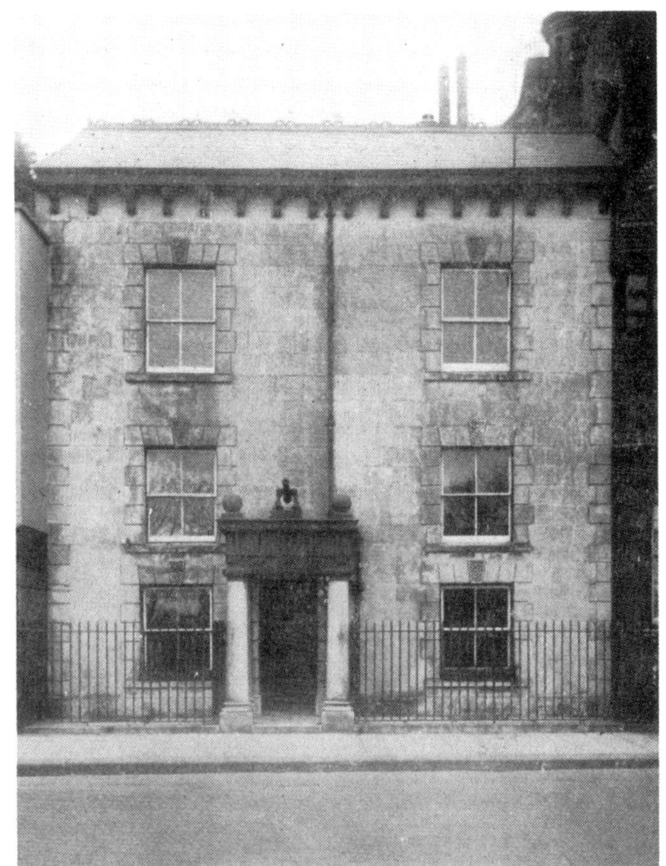

Trefalgar House.

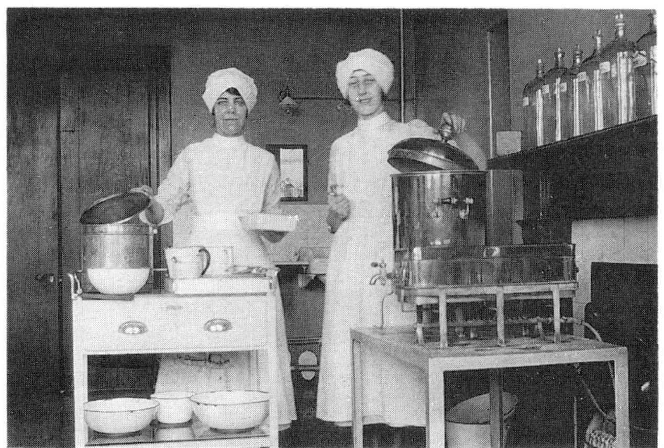

Sterilising room.

Until this could be arranged special appeals had to continue. Buying " Trafalgar House" featured often in financial statements as it would need considerable alterations from the days when it was owned by Mrs Matcham, Lord Nelson's sister. Lord Nelson was said to have met Lady Hamilton there when he was in Portsmouth.

Apart from its position next to the hospital one of the main attractions was the garden. This would give an outside play area for the children so getting them out of the ward into the fresh air.

The need for an X-ray machine had now become urgent so that was added to the shopping list. One unusual fund raising idea was a fair opened by the Mayor in Bransbury Park. The proprietor Mr Studt handed over a cheque for £1,580 so the show must have been well patronised. There were no expenses as these were met by the organisers. Another £1,500 was raised by Portsmouth and Southsea Round Table.

It does seem that a constant emphasis was put on money raising but the voluntary hospitals were completely self supporting and had to rely on the generosity of the local community. Whenever a cottage hospital opened in a district, the contributions from that area decreased. Any hope of planning ahead was out of the question; it was a very hand-to-mouth existence.

However the money was raised for both projects. The X-ray facility was ready for use in January 1938 and was demonstrated by the senior radiologist of Portsmouth, Dr Beverley Steeds-Bird. The nurses home was opened by Lord Horder in November the same year. It had accommodation for twenty-four nurses, ten maids, one porter and a cook. There was also a suite for the matron. With the old home now empty a start was made to convert it into wards. When this was finished there were sixty-three beds available.

Shortly after the outbreak of war, the hospital suffered its first air raid damage. The new nurses home was hit by fire bombs in August 1940. The wards were not touched but the home suffered considerably. On January 10th 1941 it received a direct hit and some of the lower

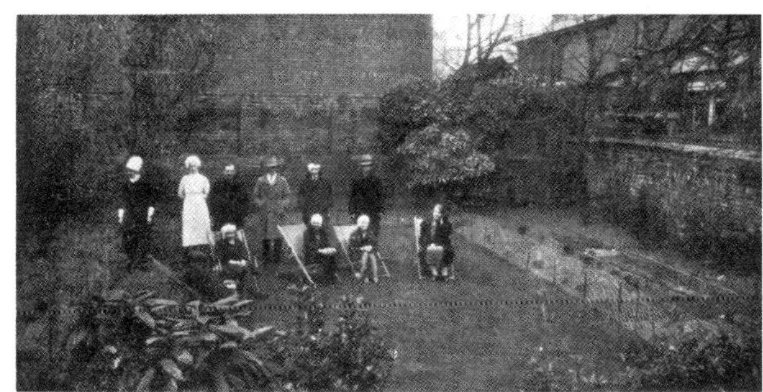

Garden which was bought with "Trefalgar House."

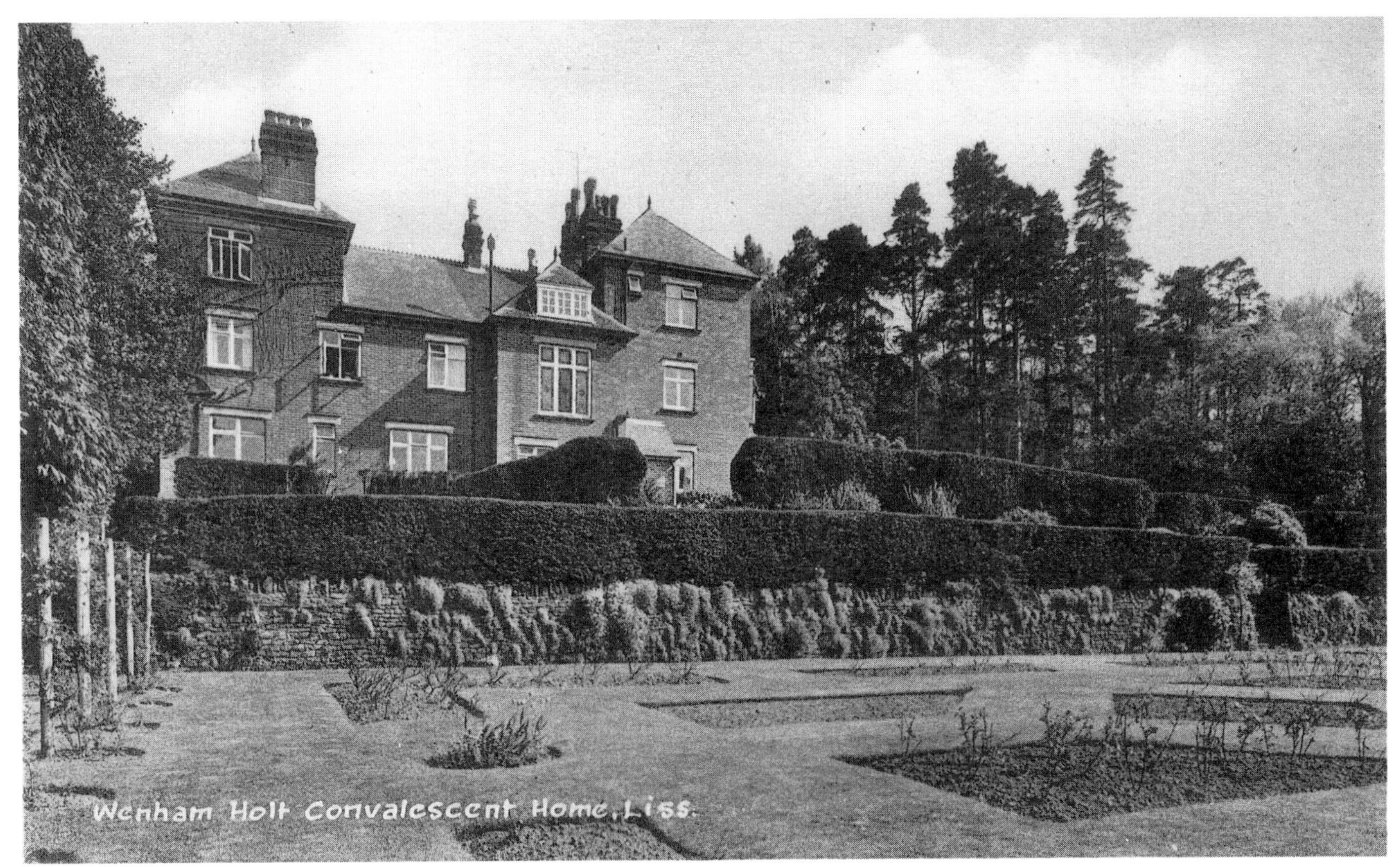

"Wenham Holt" Hill Brow Liss. Eye and Ear Hospital 1941/44.

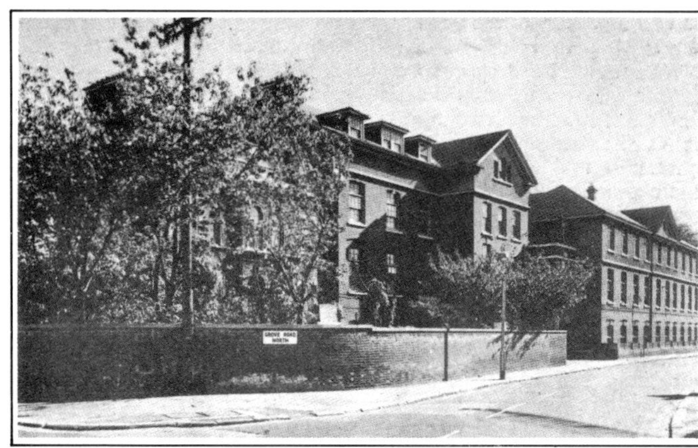

Eye and Ear Hospital, Grove Road North, Southsea. 1944/70.

walls of the hospital were destroyed. Fortunately all the patients and staff were in the shelters in the basement. Although the raids were still going on the patients were taken to a safer place nearby and none of them had so much as a scratch.

One member of staff, Major Webb the hospital secretary, was not as lucky. Yet in spite of having injuries both to his arm and his leg he organised the evacuation. The senior surgeon Mr Scott Ridout drove through the raid to the hospital and he was able to take Major Webb to a nearby nursing home where his wounds were dressed.

By now all the 'phones were out of order and the conditions had become too bad for driving to be possible. The two men walked to the Guildhall where they made alternative arrangements for the patients.

Next day corporation buses took them to the Royal West Sussex Hospital at Chichester. The raids were still continuing and shortly after the buses left, a further incendiary raid set fire to what was left

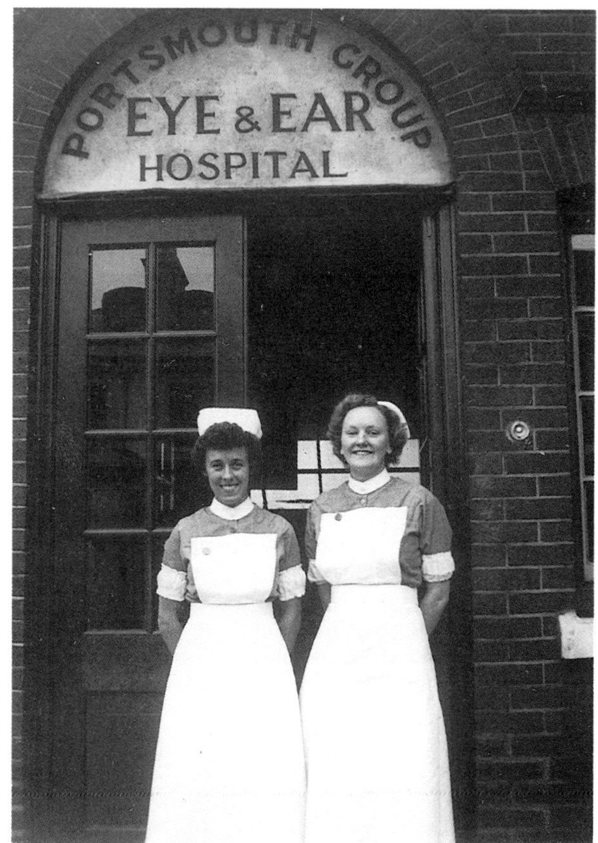

Nurses Perry and Puddick outside Grove Road entrance.

of the hospital and it became a total wreck.

It must have been a terrible blow to see all those years of work and planning destroyed in two days but there were many things to do and no time for regrets. The Rowsley Nursing Home in Kent Road was vacant and had room for twenty-four patients. Within sixteen days it was opened as a temporary hospital.

And it was indeed a temporary hospital for within six weeks that too was damaged by fire. Fortunately repairs were possible and no one was injured. On the following April there was another raid but this time the buildings were so badly damaged it was impossible to continue to house patients there. The out-patients department was still intact and clinics were held there for some time.

Within eleven weeks the patients were again rehoused. Wenham Holt, Hill Brow, Liss was brought and it remained the home of the Eye and Ear until 1944. Being twenty-five miles from Portsmouth was a great disadvantage but in another way it was a good thing as it was well north of the bombing. By 1943 the raids were less frequent so it was decided to return. In 1944 the hospital moved once more this time to a former school, the Convent of the Holy Cross, in Grove Road South, Southsea. This building is no longer standing as it has been demolished to make way for a block of flats.

As usual during the war, hospitals helped each other as far as was possible. Until the Eye and Ear returned, all adenoid and tonsil patients were looked after at St Mary's Hospital and when Rowsley was closed completely the out-patients were seen at the Royal with the Eye and Ear Staff Nurse J. Bailey in charge as she had been since the days im Pembroke Road.

Another thing all hospitals had in common was their active social life. In the twenties and thirties the Eye and Ear staff went on an annual picnic. As there were not too many of them the doctors used their own transport to travel to the venue. It was a truly family affair. Naturally there were usual parties at Christmas. Christmas Day was devoted to the patients and on Boxing Day the staff celebrated. The

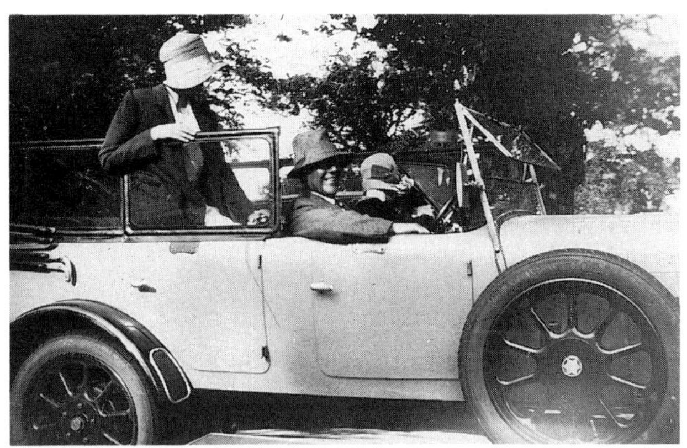

Going to the annual picnic.

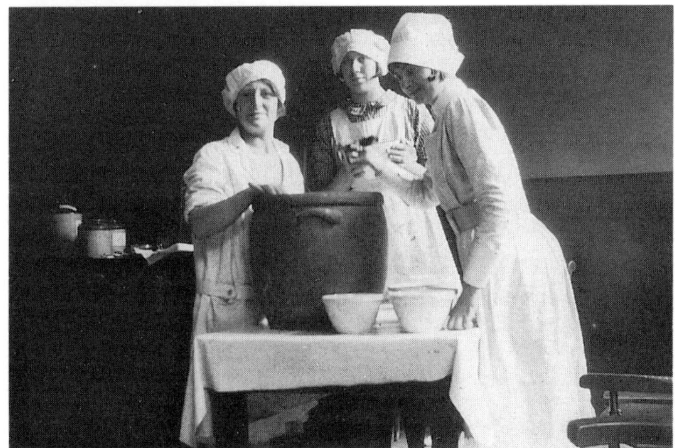

Stirring the puddings.

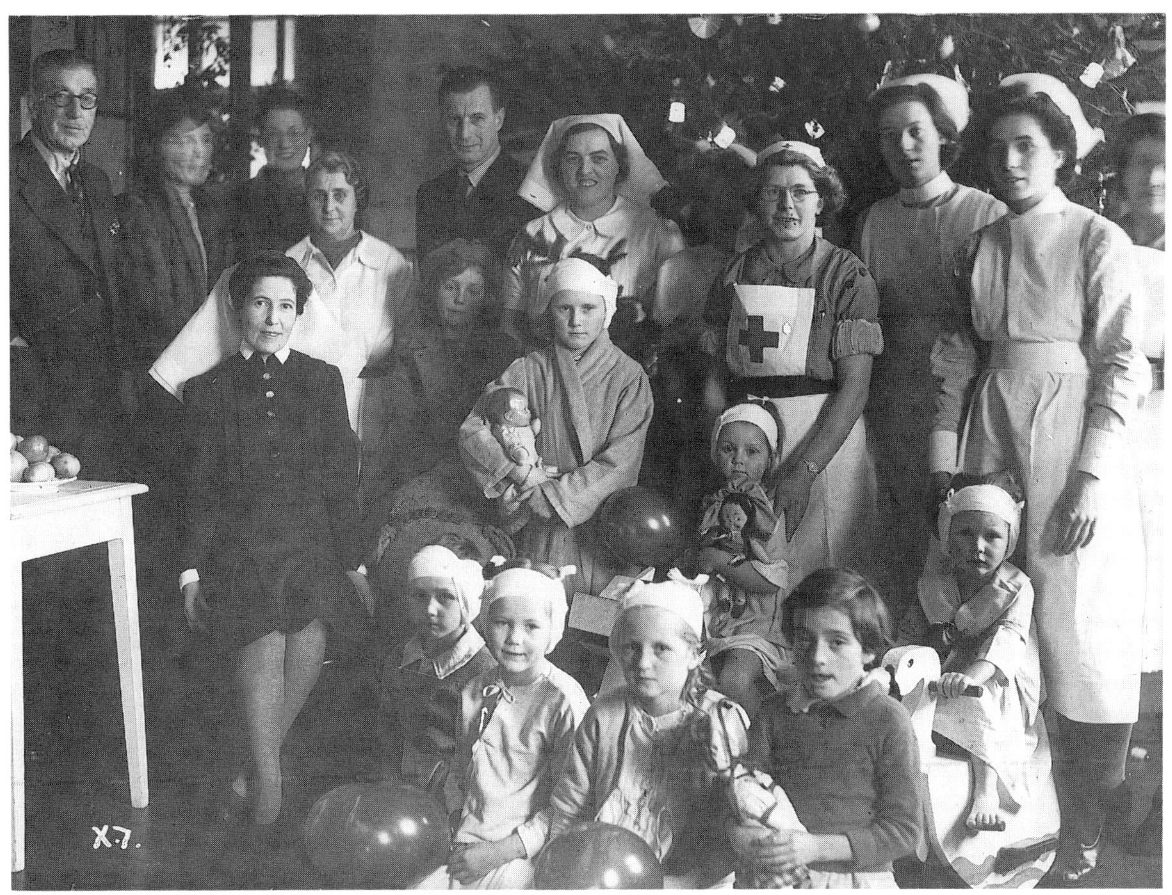

Ward ready for Christmas.

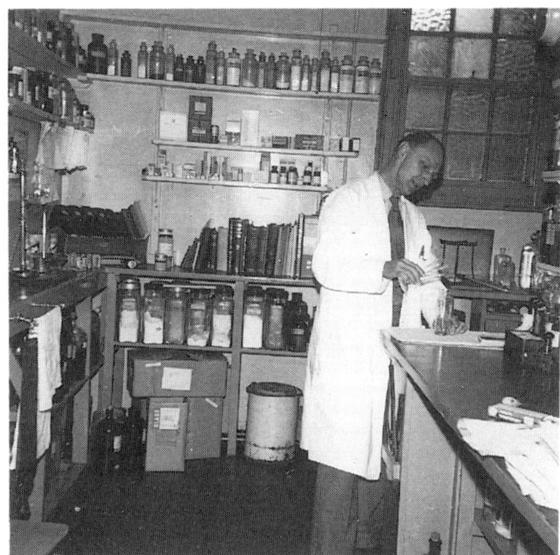

Dispensary at Grove Road.

war did not curtail either the enjoyment or the decorations in the wards. The puddings had their traditional stir in the kitchens and the turkey was carved by one of the surgeons.

The return to Portsmouth and settling into the convent did cause anxiety for some of the staff, though it did not appear to worry the patients. One night a small boy asked for a glass of water. The nurse was sidetracked by another patient and it was some time before she remembered the child. When she got back to him he was no longer interested as he said a lady in grey had already given him one. There was no one on the staff of that description but more than one nurse had seen her and were disturbed. A great many hospitals have a well authenticated ghost but they are friendly in their way. They always seem to appear when a nurse has committed a sin of omission, like forgetting a small boy who was thirsty. It was the first time a ghost had joined the staff of the Eye and Ear so they concluded she must have either come from the convent or from Ivanhoe, the house next door which had also been leased to the hospital.

In 1945 with the war over, the future had to be settled. It had to be decided if they should stay at the convent or go into new premises in the Pendragon Hotel which had formerly been used by the Admiralty. Two architects went to the Pendragon and thought it would be very difficult to redesign as a hospital. A third who was consulted thought otherwise. But the decision was soon resolved — a shortage of building material finally tipped the balance.

It was arranged that they would stay at the convent until the school needed it again. Then the school bought other buildings at Stakes Hill Road, Waterlooville and the old building was up for sale.

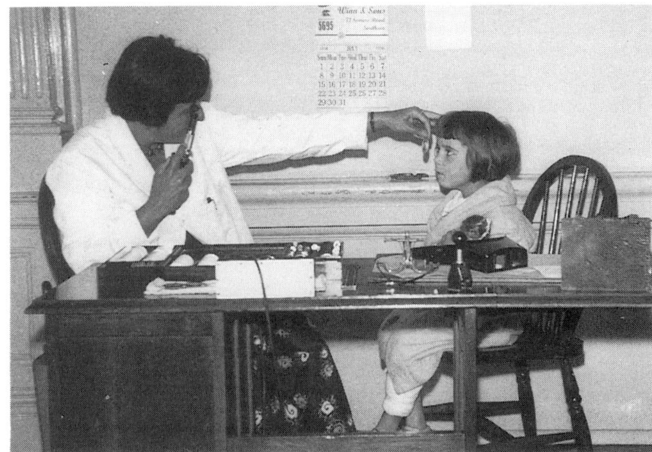

Eye Dept. Grove Road.

The arrangements were completed and the convent and Ivanhoe were bought for £57.000. It was hoped that all necessary alterations would be finished before the National Health Service took over in 1948 but there were delays. In spite of this the committee said that they had every right to feel satisfied that when on July 5th 1948 they handed over to the state, the hospital would be freehold premises, free from debt, which with investments represented a capital value of £100,000. A great deal of money achieved after sixty-five years of constant fund raising and careful housekeeping.

From 1946 onwards changes were taking place. Nurses were sent from St Mary's for three months of specialised training. Out-patients attendances increased by 4,000 over the year before. The bed situation was becoming more acute with the tonsil and adenoid waiting list reaching an unacceptable level. In March 1948 additional beds were available and five hundred cases were cleared in six weeks.

Previously there had been a relay radio service for in-patients but now this was replaced by separate head phones. Another improvement for local people came about in 1950. Up to then it had been necessary to go to Southampton to have a hearing aid fitted; now it could be done at the Eye and Ear. The demand was so great it was necessary to get two full time fitters based in Portsmouth. Soon the Isle of Wight came into the scheme and two visits a week were made to the Royal Isle of Wight County Hospital, Ryde. Portsmouth was now a full distribution centre where medical aids were stocked and also received for repairs.

In 1955 all 'Ear Nose and Throat' cases were transferred to Queen Alexandra, Cosham. Except for six beds kept for emergency E.N.T. cases, the whole of the Eye and Ear was used for eye patients. For the first time the beds were not fully used. It was feared this would put the hospital's continued existence at risk. In spite of this a new pharmacy department was opened in 1958

In 1963 it was announced by the Wessex Regional Hospital Board that the future of the Eye and Ear was now in doubt as a new Opthalmic

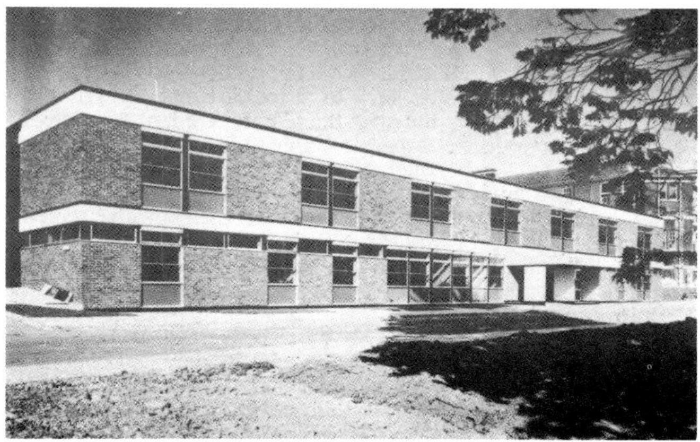

Ophthalmic Unit Queen Alexandra Hospital, Cosham.

Unit and E.N.T. Department with operating theatre was being built at Queen Alexandra.

Four years later it was decided the E.N.T. out-patients department would be moved to St Mary's as a temporary measure. So the Eye and Ear was gradually losing its identity. Soon afterwards, following eighty-five years of service it was closed. For sixty-four years it had been supported by voluntary contributions.

But Eye and Ear is still an important part of Queen Alexandra. On F level there is an eighty-six bed unit, part of which is taken up by adult and child E.N.T.; out-patients departments are on D level. Also on F level is the dental unit.

In most hospitals there is an active league of friends. After the state took over the running of the health service in 1949, there were a great many things needed by patients which only those in day-to-day contact knew about. The first fund raising meeting of the league was on June 4th 1954. Apart from the garden parties, which were always popular, the league held whist drives, darts matches, mannequin parades and concerts; anything which would raise money was tried. To be able to add to the comfort of the patient was the main aim. Some of the purchases were unusual because they came almost within the province of the state. For instance, individual thermometers for each bed and a shower for the porters room. Of course toys for the children and extras at Christmas came high on the list.

Now the League has gone. It was wound up when the work of the hospital was transferred to Queen Alexandra. Although it lasted a comparatively short time its work was greatly appreciated by the whole hospital, patients and staff alike.

In 1911, two years before the foundation stone was laid for the enlarged Eye and Ear, another hospital was opened. This time it was funded by the municipal authorities and was opened to fill a widespread need. The ground had already been bought in 1900. This was the five acres which were used to erect huts for the care of Small Pox victims.

In 1911 arrangements were made for these patients elsewhere and the area was used to build a sanatorium. This was the Langstone Hospital for the treatment of early tuberculosis. The site can easily be traced today by following the railings which are stamped with the Portsmouth coat-of-arms. The ground runs along the shore line of Langstone Harbour, right at the end of Locksway Road, Milton. The original buildings are still there but are now privately owned. There have been many houses built around them since the hospital was closed.

When it was opened on September 11th 1911, there were six beds, three for women and three for men. By the 30th there were four more and still later one more was added. By the 11th of October the first patient had been discharged, beds were constantly occupied the usual length of stay being about eleven weeks.

It was only possible to admit early cases as the accommodation was not suitable for more advanced conditions. The ward had to serve as dining room, recreation, smoking and living room. In these conditions it was realised an impossible situation would arise should both relatively fit and very ill patients be treated. No one was refused admission but those who were able contributed to their keep.

For the more severely ill there were forty-eight beds in the Portsea Island Infirmary, now St Mary's Hospital. Later there were two blocks in the Infectious Diseases Hospital, now St Mary's East Wing.

Another type of admission were those whose extremely carious teeth excluded them from any other sanatorium. Until the condition was cleared up they remained at Langstone because they had such an excellent reputation for a speedy response to treatment. As soon as they were well enough the teeth were atttended to and the patient admitted to another institution nearer to their home.

There was the usual cry for more beds. It was decided the ideal size would be twenty-four beds and a request was put in for more accommodation. The beds granted never matched the figure hoped for so no doubt when an extra eight were allowed they were well pleased.

In 1913 changes were made to the wards; balconies were added, protected by canvas awnings with doors leading into the wards. Beds which were put out there by day could be returned to the ward at night. There was now room for seven women and twelve men. In very cold weather these arrangements presented some difficulties. They were overcome to everyone's satisfaction. There were huts in the grounds and though they were far less comfortable than the wards the men were very happy to sleep there.

The reason for this apparently noble self sacrifice on the part of the men was given by a former patient. The men liked the huts because they were far enough away from the main building. They could slip out in the evening and over to the local for a pint with a good chance of getting there and back unseen. The other customers and the landlord kept an eye on the door and let them know if any member of staff was about.

A fair proportion of the patients did not feel really ill and boredom was one of the main difficulties to be overcome. This same patient

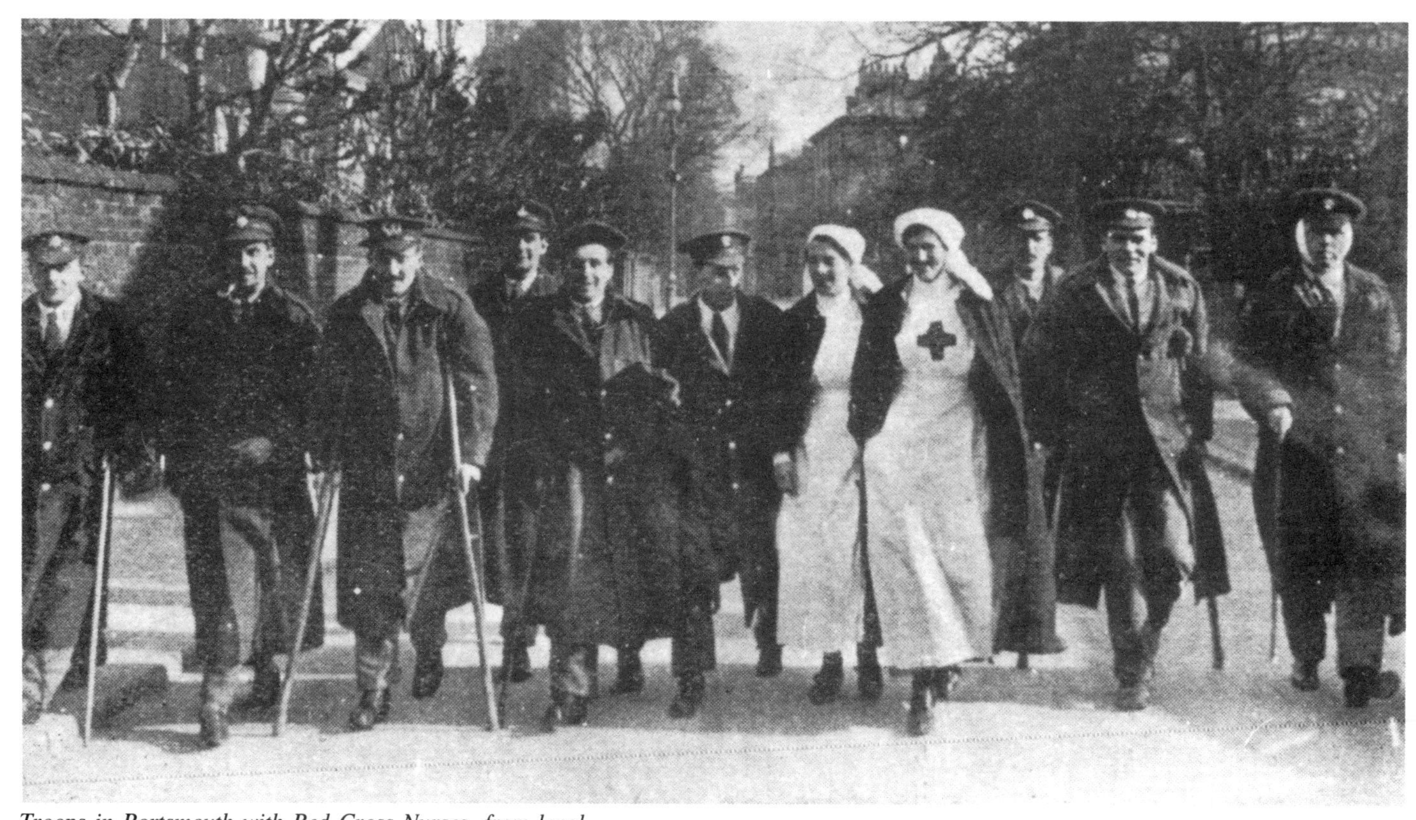

Troops in Portsmouth with Red Cross Nurses, from local Hospitals.

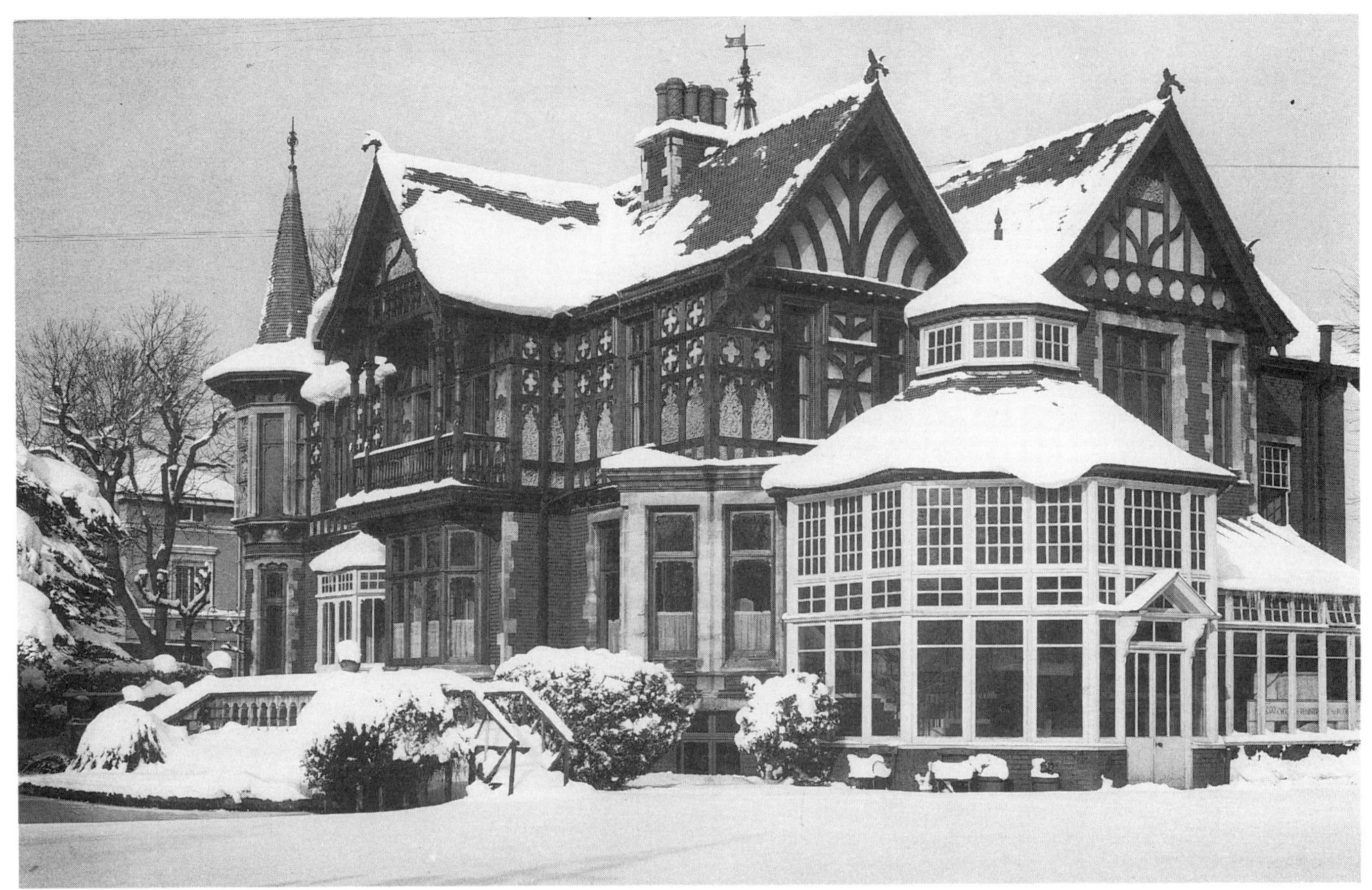

''Brankesmere'' under snow.

tells of the conversation she had with the artist Edward King when he was painting by Langstone shore. He was a patient at St James' Hospital and she enjoyed hearing about his life before he was ill. She found him to be a charming man and he obviously liked talking to her.

In 1919 Beach Lodge was opened. This was formerly the gardener's cottage which was altered to accommodate ten children. This number was reduced to nine when it was found a room was needed for the staff.

The hospital worked in conjunction with the Infectious Disease Hospital. Patients were often admitted there for special treatment or operations. Returning to Locksway Road to complete their stay before being discharged.

The hospital continued to be used until about 1951. The exact time of its closure is not clear but there are no further references to it in the accounts of the Ministry of Health meetings after 1950. No doubt new drugs used in the treatment of tuberculosis and a greater knowledge of the care of the patients reduced the incidence of the disease. In any case by now there were enough beds in the Infectious Disease Hospital.

Before giving an account of the four large hospitals in Portsmouth it would be interesting to show how the medical services managed during two world wars. During the 1914/18 war all the hospitals were to some extent involved and there were also smaller units in schools and large private houses. There was a great deal of work going on in Portsmouth in support of the war effort.

One large house which today is used by the Welfare Services was a 130-bed hospital. Between the wars it was a school and during the last war the police headquarters were based there. Now it is the offices of Portsmouth Area 3 Social Services Department.

"Branksmere" was built by Henry Jones for Sir John Brickwood, the same firm which built the laundry at St Mary's Hospital in 1895. The two buildings could not be more different. "Branksmere" has a slightly Tudor look about it and is embellished with turrets and gables. Inside there are enormous carved fireplaces and wood panelling

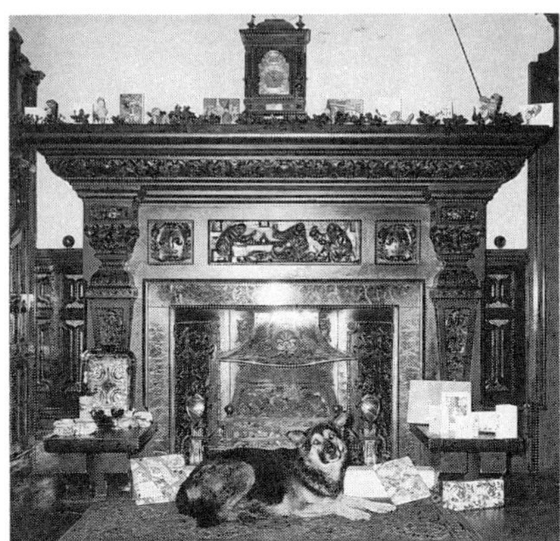

Interior of "Brankesmere" during the last war.

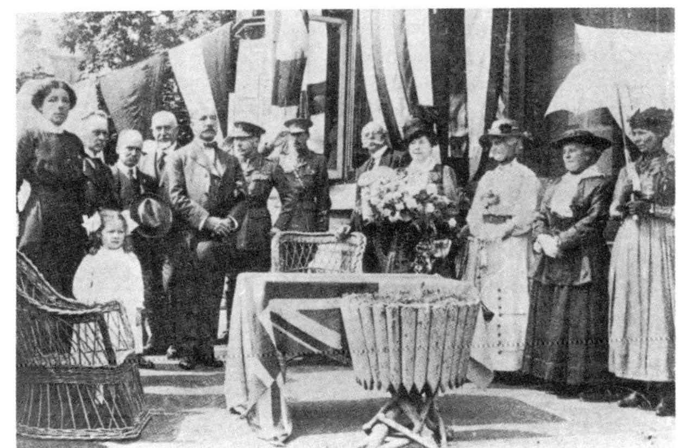

"Brankesmere" 14/18 war.

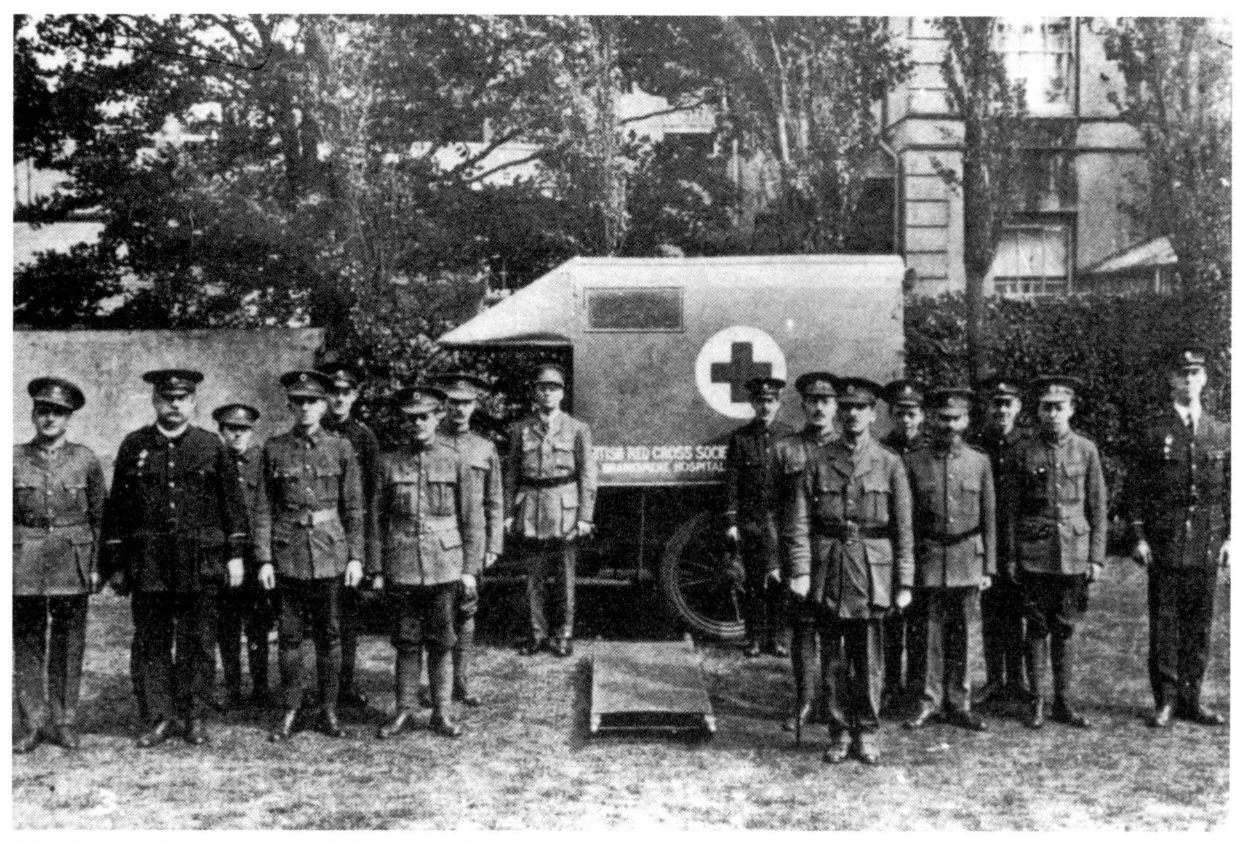

''Brankesmere'' with troops and Clement-Talbot ambulance.

everywhere. Although there was extensive damage around the area during the last war, the building came through unscathed and can be seen from Kent Road near St Judes Church.

The building was lent by the owner to the Red Cross. Apart from an initial government grant it was self-supporting, funds being raised locally. There was also a Clement Talbot motor-ambulance attached to the hospital which was lent by Mr Cecil Greenhill. Apart from this gentleman, the main running of the unit seemed to be in the hands of single ladies. The honorary secretary was Miss M. Ellis M.B.E., the quartermaster Miss Crookenden and Miss Stroud and Miss Ellis were the honorary dispensers.

The size of the house can be judged by the fact that there were seventy beds in the house itself. A further sixty beds were in tents in the grounds. In all 2,385 wounded were cared for during the war. The surroundings must have come as a welcome change after the mud and horror of the trenches.

Another house lent for the duration was "Oaklands" in Kingston Crescent. It was owned by Mr Frank Bevis and in this case it was run by the V.A.D. (Volunteer Aid Detachment). It must have been a smaller house as there were only thirty-eight beds but even so it was a good size. In all a thousand patients were nursed there so the contribution to the war effort was considerable. There is no sign of the house today and it is not known when it was demolished.

Local schools were also taken over. The boys and the girls secondary schools in Fawcett Road were both used and there were one hundred and fifty beds in Francis Avenue School. When the beds allocated by the hospitals are added to this, the extent of casualty work going on in the area can be imagined.

Most of St Mary's, three wards of the Royal and facilities at both the Eye and Ear and the Infectious Diseases Hospital were also used for war wounded. Added to this list was naturally the military hospital on the hill, Queen Alexandra, plus for a short while, St James Hospital, Milton.

During the Second World War the position was different. Two of the hospitals were built next to a large installation each of which was a prime target for enemy action; the Royal next to the Dockyard and the Eye and Ear next to the Victoria Barracks. They were both extensively damaged and both St James' and St Marys' had their share of trouble.

At the start of the war, most casualty work was involved with civilian wounded. When the Royal was so badly hit that it was no longer possible to admit patients. St James' allocated ninety beds which were staffed by nurses from the Royal, so the hospital was still able to function. These beds were used as an emergency medical unit and it became a clearing station for battle casualties who were flown from the various fields of conflict in Europe. There were also a few beds still kept for routine admissions.

The service patients were given treatment, X-rays etc. and were often transferred the same day. The first question the men asked was "How long shall I be here?" then "Where am I anyway?," hoping that by some miracle they were near home and there would be visits from the family. Each intake did have a visitor however short their stay. A small Roman Catholic priest arrived as if by magic and went around the wards at great speed with the cry "Any R.Cs any R.Cs?" The eagerness with which hands went up showed his presence was welcomed.

Sometimes a German P.O.W. got mixed up with the rest but a local schoolmaster sorted out that problem by acting as interpreter. Another snag was how to send X-rays with the patients.

Staff Nurse Thompson produced a rather unorthodox solution. There were no quick dryers or automatic processing machines. So the wet films were hung up on lines wherever space could be found, secured by safety pins, then hung in the ambulance to finish drying. Or, when the supply of safety pins ran out, the still wet film was rolled in a piece of (it was hoped) non-stick material.

Only the in-patients were transferred to St James' after the raids in 1942. the out-patients departments remained in the original buildings. The X-ray department had thick blast proof walls built to cover the windows and the dark room which had a flat roof, was well protected by sand bags. The staff were taken there daily from Foster Hall, the hall of residence at the teachers training college, in Locksway Road, to staff casualty and out-patients.

Accounts of the actual damage to the hospitals is included in the history of the hospitals themselves. The first to be built of the four large hospitals was the Royal Portsmouth, Portsea and Gosport Hospital, later known as the Royal Portsmouth Hospital. And no account would be complete without a brief review of the life of the founder.

Dr W.C. Engledue was born in Portsea in 1813. He was articled to Dr Porter of Portsea who realised he had an outstanding pupil and arranged for his admission to the Edinburgh Medical School. Within two years he was allowed to sit his final examinations, a concession which was quite without precedent. At the age of twenty-one he was elected president of the Royal Medical Society of Edinburgh.

After staying in Scotland for only a year he returned to Portsea leaving a highly lucrative practice to do so. From that time he devoted his life to improving the lot of the poor of his native town.

He immediately put forward the idea of adding beds to the Portsmouth and Portsea Dispensary which had been started thirteen years before in St Georges Square. This idea was rejected by his fellow physicians who were afraid it would harm their practices. In fact they were so upset by the whole thing they ostracised him even to the extent of refusing to work or consult with him. He was obviously a brilliant young man and this lack of contract with his fellow practitioners must have been a great loss not only to the patients but to the medical profession.

Fortunately it did not deter him. He was determined that there would be a hospital in Portsea. Helped by a substantial cheque from Mr T.E. Owen the Mayor-elect, the foundation stone of the Royal Portsmouth Portsea and Gosport Hospital was laid on September 17th 1847, fourteen years after Dr Engledue's return.

A life devoted to the people of Portsea ended sadly. When working in the hospital he contracted erysipelas and died at the age of forty-five on December 30th 1857.

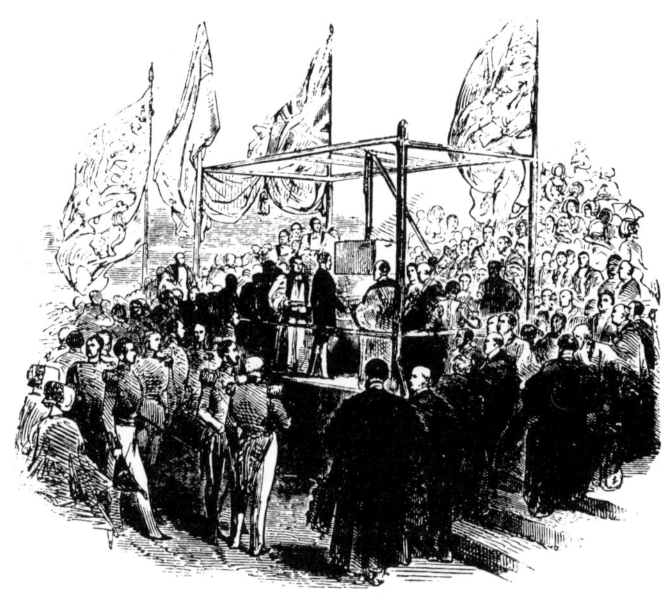

Prince Albert laying foundation stone of the Royal Hospital 1847.

The ceremony of laying of the foundation stone was a great affair. It was not only reported in the local paper but in the *Illustrated London News* in which it was given substantial coverage in the issue of October 2nd 1847. The reason for this could have been presence of the Queens Consort H.R.H. Prince Albert who no doubt added greatly to the importance of the occasion.

He arrived at the Albert Pier, Portsea in the "Fire Queen" to the sound of the band of the 52nd Regiment playing the National Anthem. A salute was fired from the battery and from the "Victory" whose yards were manned. He was escorted to Admiral Sir Charles Ogle's carriage and from there to the hospital site.

The whole route was lined with cheering crowds and there was accommodation for about a thousand to sit around the platform on stands which were bedecked with flags. As all these spectators were ticket holders, the *Illustrated London News* reporter was right when he observed: "The amount taken must have been considerable." So the hospital got off to both a good ceremonial and financial start.

Many local worthies appeared on the list of distinguished guests. Lord George Lennox, Mr W. Grant, chairman of the management committee, the deputy chairman Dr Scott and the secretary Mr Ford. Also Colonel Lewis, Captain Chads and Major White.

Among the clergy was the Dean of Winchester, the Vicar of Portsmouth the Reverend J.P. M'Ghie and the Warden of Winchester College. There were also the aldermen and councillors of Portsmouth Council. The Mayor, Benjamin Bramble read a congratulatory letter on behalf of the council. In fact by the sound of it they all had a simply splendid time.

In his reply to the letter the Prince said:

"I have received with much pleasure your address. I very willingly consent to lay the first stone of the hospital in your borough, for nothing can be more gratifying to my feelings than to be able to promote and encourage the useful and charitable institutions of the country; and no undertaking can be more deserving of such a description than that which provide refuge, assistance and medical skill for suffering in the combined misfortune of poverty and sickness."

The architects Owen and Livesay were unable to be there so the contractor Mr Absolem supervised the actual laying of the stone. Afterwards Mr W. Grant handed His Royal Highness a silver gilt trowel. The ceremony was concluded with prayers led by the Warden of Winchester College the Reverend R.S. Barter.

Less than eighteen months later on January 2nd 1849 the new hospital was opened. The opening ceremony was preceeded by Divine Service which took place at St Thomas's Church in the morning. The sermon was preached by the Bishop of Winchester who took as his text: "I was a stranger and you took me in."

The hospital cost £2,310 to build so the collection which came to £120 was quite a considerable donation to the hospital funds. The official opening in the afternoon was a fairly quiet affair. It was attended only by those who were directly concerned with the running of the institution. The Bishop of Winchester was there in his capacity as President, the Reverend Alex Lowery as the hospital chaplain, Dr T.P. Simpson M.D. honorary houseman, six doctors from the borough, all honorary medical officers and the members of the committee.

An announcement was made by the commmittee to the effect that during any outbreak of cholera no ticket would be needed to come for treatment; anyone could come. The hospital was declared open by the chairman.

The threat of cholera was a very real one. Since his return to Portsea, Dr Engledue had been campaigning for an improvement in the water supply. There were two waterworks companies, The Portsea Island and the Farlington, and there was constant trouble between them. Hoping to gain some influence on their committees he bought shares in both of them. It was an uphill task and even when they were joined in 1840 there was no peace. It was not until 1857 that pure water was available in any quantitiy. Up to the time the hospital was opened, there was a constant danger of pollution of the wells from nearby

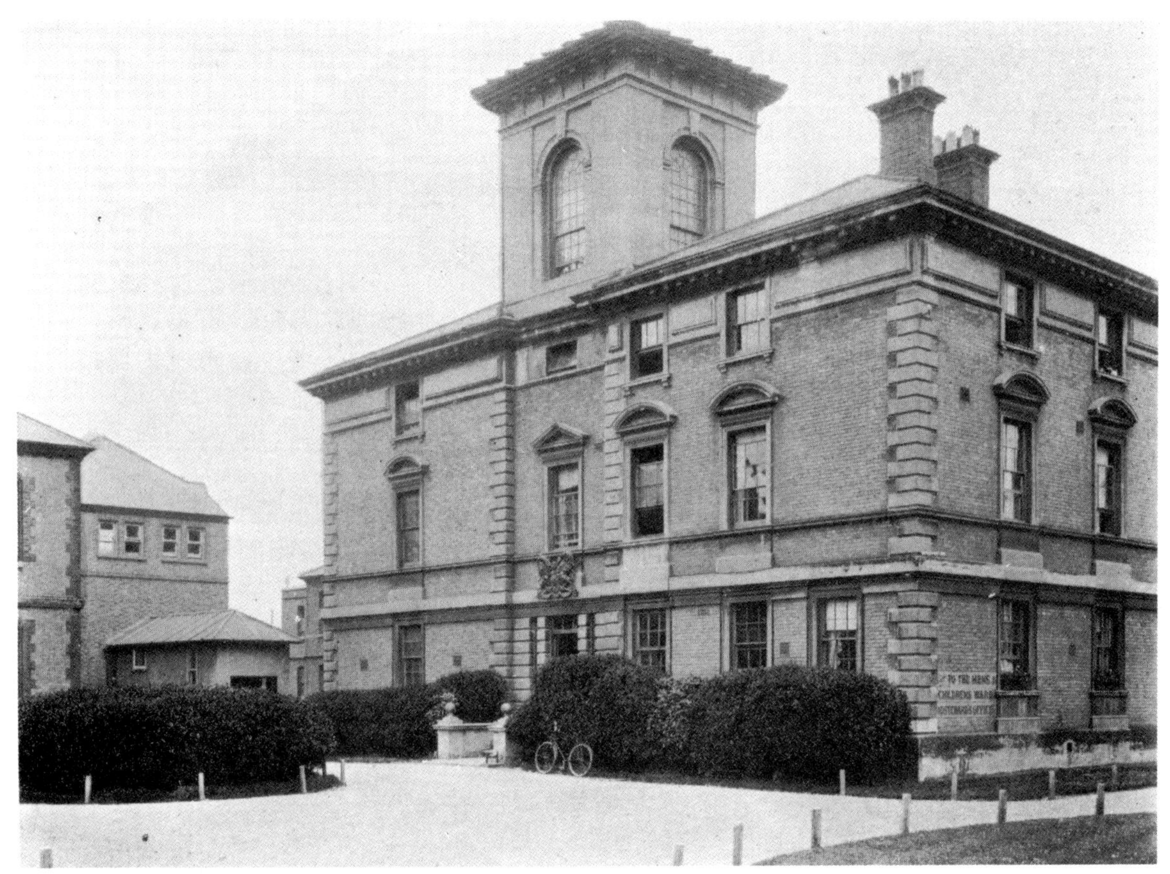

Royal Hospital 1849.

cesspits. Between August and September of that year there had been an outbreak in which six hundred and seventy-eight people had died, far worse than the previous year when one hundred and fifty were lost. On September 16th there was a day of prayer when the dockyard and all premises were closed. By November the epidemic had abated and a general thanksgiving took place. A collection amounting to £147 was given to the hospital.

Eleven years after Dr Engledue died, public baths were opened in the hospital grounds, the cost being met by public subscription. They were opened daily except Sundays from 8 a.m. till 8 p.m.; entry one shilling.

The hospital was described in the Portsmouth Council papers of March 18th 1849 as a handsome white brick building. It was built on land leased by the Board of Ordnance for a thousand years at a pepper-corn rent on the understanding that a hospital would always stand there. At first there were twelve beds and the building ran from east to west, parallel to Fitzherbert Street. The ward, waiting room, dispensary and entrance hall had a north aspect while the kitchen and operating room faced south. The lodge and entrance were a short distance from the corner of Commercial Road. There was ample room for extension both to the east and the west; this ground was soon put to good use.

At first there were three nurses with a combined salary of £31.10s per year. As the patients increased in number so did the staff. Six years later a matron was appointed at a salary of £30 a year and a resident surgeon at £80.

In 1887 the first probationer nurse was accepted for training, the course to be spread over three years. At the same time a department was established to provide trained nurses to care for patients in their own homes. There were strict rules laid down as to the nurses' conduct when on duty outside the hospital. They had to have seven consecutive rest hours away from the sick room every twenty-four. No meals would be taken in the sick room or with the servants. In addition the nurse would take at least one hour of exercise out of doors each day and attend Divine Service every Sunday.

In 1895 the convalescent fund was started by an anonymous donor who contributed £1,500. A further £500 was given by Sir John Baker M.P. and other contributions added another £265. At this point it was decided that rather than build a separate home it would be invested so that existing institutions could be used. So again the hospital care was extended outside the hospital itself.

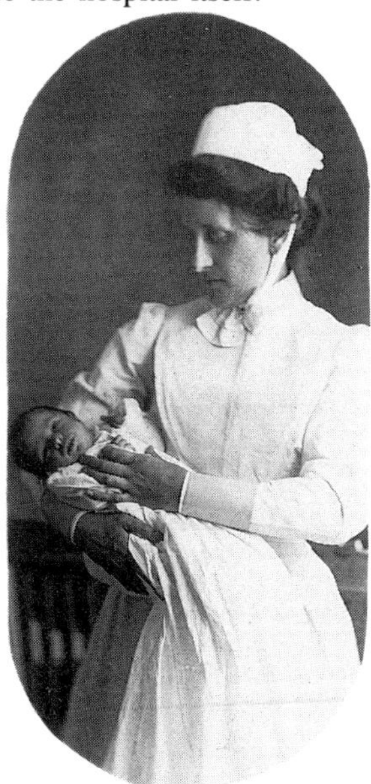

Nurse Sophia Tarrant. One of the hospital nurses working privately. 1911.

The hospital was enlarged at a remarkable speed. The population of Portsmouth in 1849 was only 70,000 so there must have been great enthusiasm on the part of the fund raisers.

Within a year three more wards were built and in 1868 the Baring Block was opened. In the first instance this was used as a childrens ward but later it was used for surgical cases. It was named as a memorial to Sir F.J. Baring, first Lord Northbrook who for thirty years was Member of Parliament for Portsmouth. Still there were not nearly enough beds and in times of emergency it was often necessary to put mattresses on the floor for extra patients. It is impossible to imagine the difficulties the nurses had to overcome.

In 1878 there was accommodation for fifty-six patients — fifteen male and seventeen female. Added to that were ten childrens and fourteen beds reserved for accident cases. There were also the Lock wards but these, which contained thirty beds, were used and financed by the Admiralty and closed at the end of the century.

All the wards were named after people who had been benefactors in various ways. Ogle Ward after Admiral Sir Charles Ogle C-in-C Portsmouth who had supported the hospital from its inception; Dixon Ward after Sir Charles Dixon of Stanstead, always generous with help; Thistlewyte Ward after the owner of Southwick House while Grant Ward was probably named after Mr W. Grant who was chairman of the committee of management at the time when the foundation stone was laid. There was also a long standing supporter in the Reverend Grant Vicar of Portsmouth who was chairman for fourteen years. Gilman Ward was named after the first Treasurer and Engledue after the founder. Lastly Gaslee recalled a liberal Member of Parliament in 1865 whose interest in the hospital carried on a family tradition of supporting local institutions. He was the grandson of an eminent surgeon who was Mayor of Portsmouth from 1797-1800. Although many of these names are no longer well known they were important citizens in their day.

Comparing the survey map of the original building with that of 1874, great changes have taken place with extensions westwards.

In 1888 it was decided that the local Jubilee Memorial Fund would be invested with a view to enlarge the hospital in the very near future. The sum of £3,209 16s 7d was put aside for the purpose. On May 1st, 1888 some new wards were opened by the Bishop of Winchester. The next year an isolation building with four beds was added and in 1891 the opening of a new laundry costing £500 was a very necessary addition. In 1897 £1,000 was spent on a new nurses home with twenty separate rooms.

Even with these improvements there was still not enough accommodation to meet the growing needs of the area. At a meeting convened by the Mayor Mr G. Couzens on January 19th 1897 it was decided that the Queens Jubilee Fund would be entirely devoted to the building of a new block of wards.

There was so much interest that it was arranged that the Free Mart Fair would be revived. It had been abolished in 1847 because it was considered to be "a great danger to the public peace and morals". Before that date the fairs had been held in Portsmouth over a period of six hundred years.

The Jubilee version was a very well organised affair. It was held in the old town hall in the High Street for three days (July 6th 7th and 8th) under Royal Patronage, a fact which was printed in large capital letters on the posters. The names of the Duke and Duchess of Connaught, H.R.H. Princess Louise and the Duke and Duchess of York showed that the fund raisers of those days knew their job.

The names on the posters were also reassuring to anyone who had heard of the past reputation of the Fairs. It was said they encouraged pickpockets, human monstrosities and other abominations. Surely this would be impossible under such a distinguished umbrella.

It was advertised with the following words: "This revival of the Free Mart Fair in 1897 has been designed in aid of the new building fund of the Royal Portsmouth and Gosport Hospital and all who do business at the fair, or take pleasure in the entertainment so liberally provided will have the comforting assurances they are helping in a noble cause."

There would have been much to see, including wax works, phonographs, electrical apparatus and X-ray equipment. Unfortunately in 1897 the dangerous properties of the latter were not fully understood. It can only be hoped they were not too enthusiastically demonstrated. In addition to the exhibits there were concerts to enjoy and a palmist was installed in the magistrates room. And a very good place to put her too.

So with Royalty, the Mayor and Mayoress, the Commander-in-Chief and two local Members of Parliament as sponsors, the Fair was well and truly launched. It proved to be a considerable boost to the Jubilee Fund. By the end of the year £15,000 had been raised from various projects.

It was decided a start could be made on the buildings, first on two wards with the others to follow as soon as the money was available. The foundation stone was laid by the Duke of Connaught on August 7th 1897. The complete block was opened by the Duke and Duchess of York on March 1st 1899, by which time there were two blocks, not one as originally planned.

The new buildings were sited to run from north to south so avoiding the north facing aspect which was one of the disadvantages of the old. As the new wards were ready, the old ones were gradually phased out, although the building was still used. The male ward was turned into the X-ray department and the female ward became the kitchen and stores. The matron's rooms and the administration offices were also a part of the old building. These were destroyed during the air raid of April 27th 1941.

Unfortunately when the administration offices went so did the board room and with it the portraits of many of Portsmouth's most able men, men who had been remembered when the wards in the original hospital had been named; Admiral Sir Charles Ogle, Mr Gilman, Mr Charles Dixon and Dr Engledue and many others whose interest helped enormously in running the hospital and in financing it.

Admiral Sir Henry Chads and the Reverend E.P. Grant were both committee members and the Reverend Grant was also chairman for fourteen years. Canon Edgar Jacob was Vicar of Portsmouth from 1878-1896 and was largely responsible for the success of the Hospital Sunday Fund. The Reverend Cosmo Gordon Lang was also Vicar of Portsmouth before he became Archbishop of York and during his stay in the town he was a constant supporter of the institution. Three surgeons on the staff were Mr E.K. Parsons, Mr K.E. Knight and Mr H. Rundle. Mr Henry Rundle F.R.C.S. was responsible for various papers on the history of the Royal and they are useful source of information on its early years. Also remembered in the Board Room was Dr John Ward Cousins a physician who worked for the hospital for forty-eight years. Most of them were not only involved with the working of the hospital but with events in the town itself.

The two blocks which were opened by the Duke and Duchess of York in 1899 consisted of two storeys with one ward on each containing twenty beds. At the end of the wards was a separate area for baths and lavatories. According to the account given at the time: "The floors of the wards were of terrazzo masaic and nowhere is there a corner for dust to secure a foot hold." The wards were named Duchess of York, Victoria, Connaught and Albert.

As the need for extensions continued so did the fund raising. The abilities of the local people in this respect had always been extraordinary. As far back as 1849 a bazaar was held which raised £479.14.6d whilst another six years later brought in £633.2s 6d, a great deal of money for those days.

At the time of the Free Mart Fair Mr George Couzens was Mayor of Portsmouth. Eight years later in 1905 he once more had an ambitious idea to raise funds. This time he had surpassed himself. He also set a very large target, £20,000.

On July 11th, 12th, 13th and 14th of that year a Grand Trafalgar Bazaar and Exhibition was held. This time it was in the new Town Hall which had been opened in 1890. It was billed as being in aid

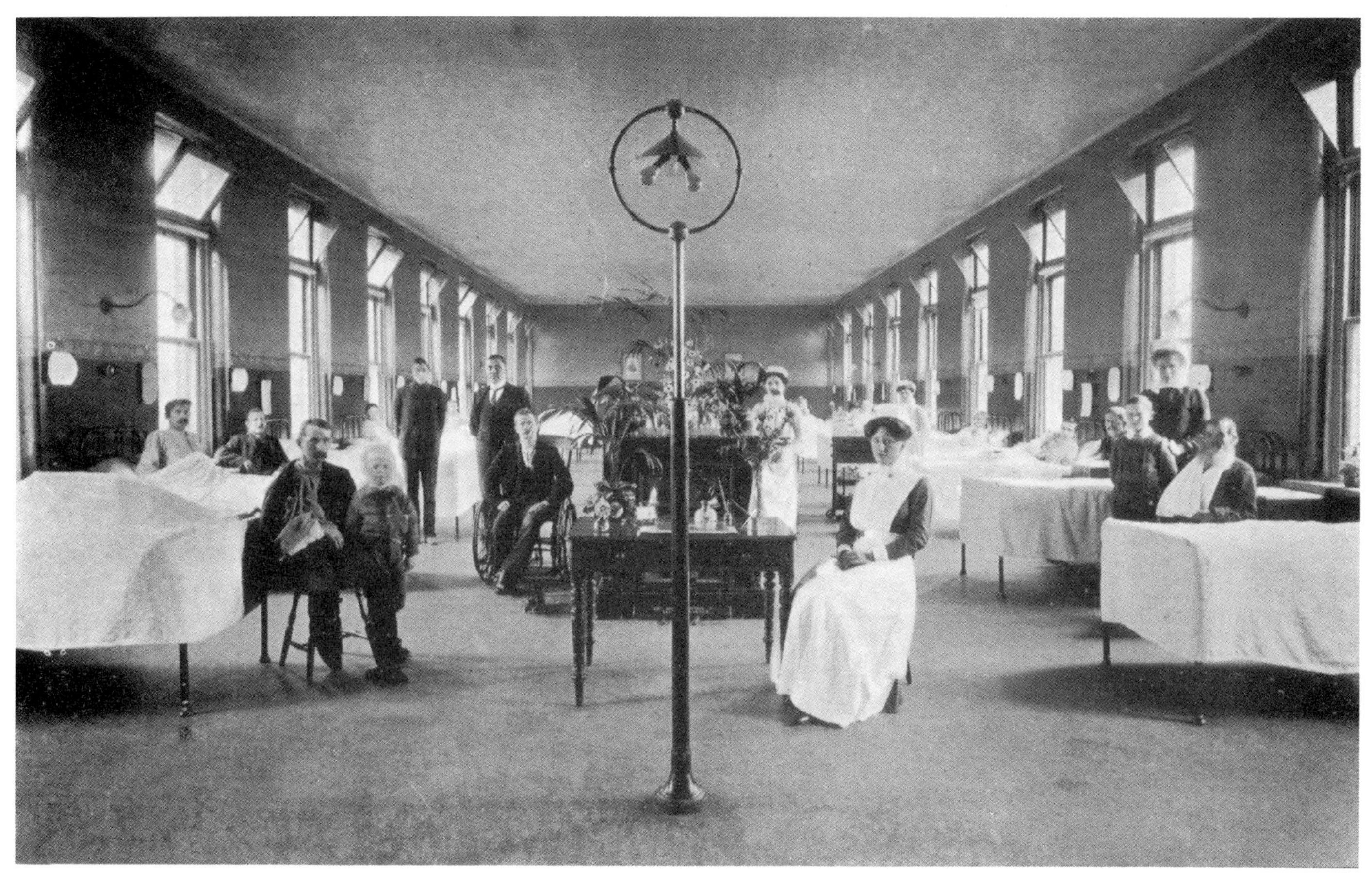

Mens Ward. New Block Royal Hospital.

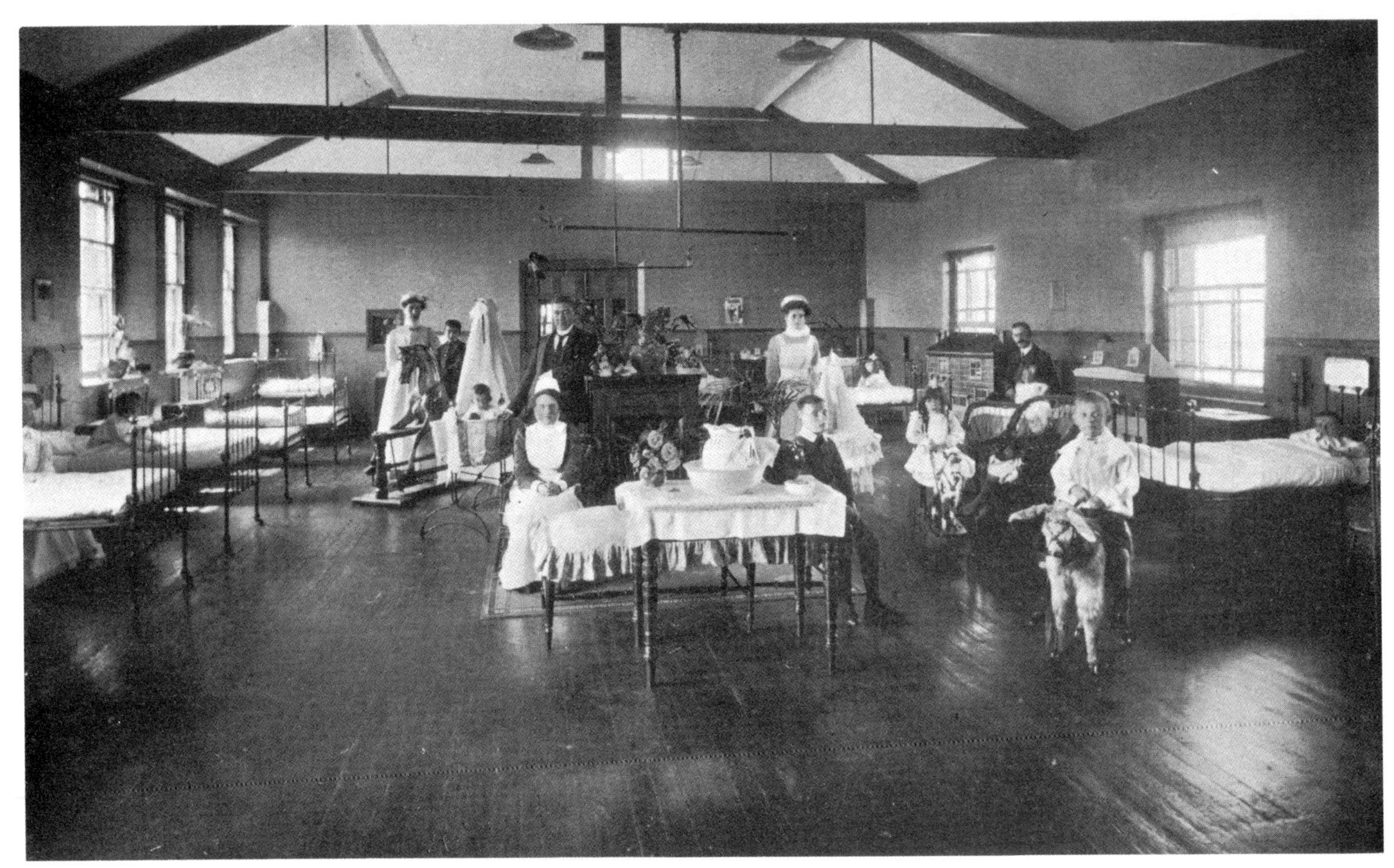

Childrens Ward. Old Block Royal Hospital.

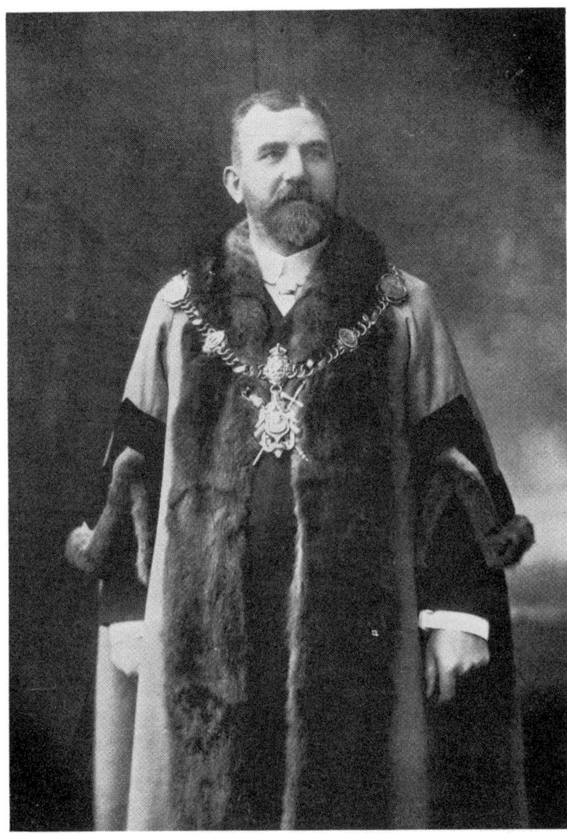

George E. Couzens. Great Fund raiser. Mayor of Portsmouth 1905.

of the Mayors Fund for the erection of a new block and operating theatre in the Royal Portsmouth, Portsea and Gosport Hospital. In the posters for the Free Mart Fair, the word Portsea was omitted from the title but now it reappeared. The entrance fee varied from 2/6 for a season ticket to 1s for half a day (5p in today's currency). That was at the start of the exhibition but for the last two days it was 6d all day. There were separate exhibitions, band concerts and theatrical entertainments for which a charge usually of 6d was made.

The official programme described twenty-seven pages of stalls and entertainments. Also a plan of the hospital with a key showing the existing parts, proposed parts and those which required completion. So the public knew what the appeal was all about.

The first page after the Mayor's introduction had three columns of closely typed names of patrons. As they were not in alphabetical order or as far as can be seen in any particular order of precedence, some people must have been offended in those very class conscious days. To make matters worse, at the end of the list were printed the words etc, etc; — not the most tactful way of ensuring that nobody was left out.

The next page was equally closely typed with the names of the general committee and the honorary secretaries of which there were eighteen, and who formed the executive committee.

The programme makes wonderful reading and gives a great insight into the lavish way things were done in Edwardian times. Most of the stalls had a theme and the stall holders dressed accordingly. The hospital stall must have been the easiest as it was run by the matron and her nurses who wore their usual uniforms. The others must have made a lovely splash of colour. There was the nautical stall where some wore blue, some red and some white. The oriental one had plenty of scope so must the Empire, Early Victorian and Romney. The cost and work which went into setting up these stalls must have been enormous but the young society ladies in the town would have had a lovely time.

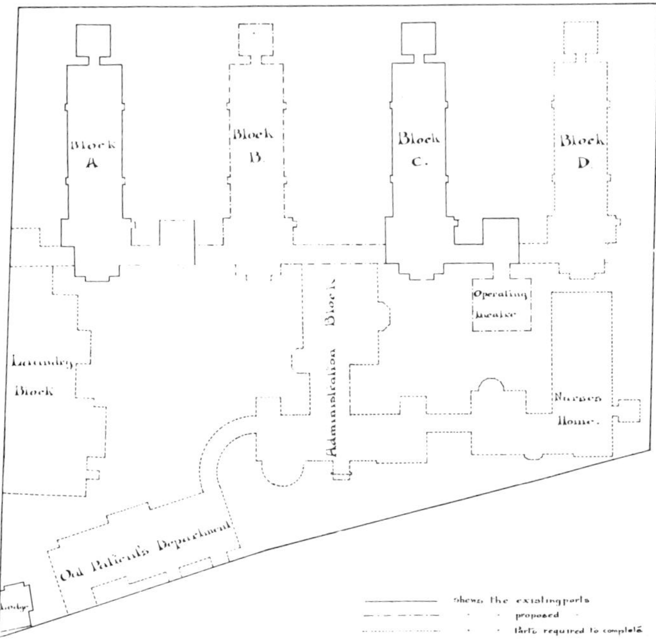

Plan for proposed alterations and additions 1905.

Most of the exhibitions, band concerts and theatrical shows cost 6d but a tableau of the Death of Nelson with commentary by Mr W.H. Saunders could be enjoyed for 3d. They even had animated photographs of the Battle of Trafalgar in the Grand Jury Room, but it cost 6d to see those. Also for 6d there was the opportunity to sign ones name on a four leaved screen "the names subsequently being rendered indelible by poker-work."

The exhibits in the electrical show were demonstrated by experts from H.M.S. Vernon and many of them sound strange today. The Röntgen Rays it was said would reveal their revealing powers. They have survived by being renamed X-rays. But the other objects have very peculiar names.

The Telautograph, the latest American invention, transmitted messages in writing. The Hermonigraph "that most laughable of scientific implements, showed its artistic abilities"; — the programmes didn't say who invented that one. At the end, an offer no Edwardian lad wanting to impress his girl could possibly refuse: — "electric shocks — strong or weak to order".

Each day the exhibition was opened by a local celebrity with the Mayor in attendance. There was a carefully posed picture of the lady on the programme and even the young ladies who presented the bouquets were mentioned. The Edwardians knew something about selling; all these names must have got rid of a great many programmes. It would have been interesting to know how much they cost but it did not say. Nor is there any record of the exact amount raised in all. The Exhibition was open from 2.20 until 10 O'clock.

As a result of the Great Trafalgar Bazaar and Exhibition, the new operating theatre was opened in 1907. It was described as having tesselated pavements and white walls completely tiled. The air was warmed and filtered and there were good electrical installations. At the time electricity was something of note.

The previous year saw the completion of the corridors which connected the two blocks. In 1908 with great financial help from Mr

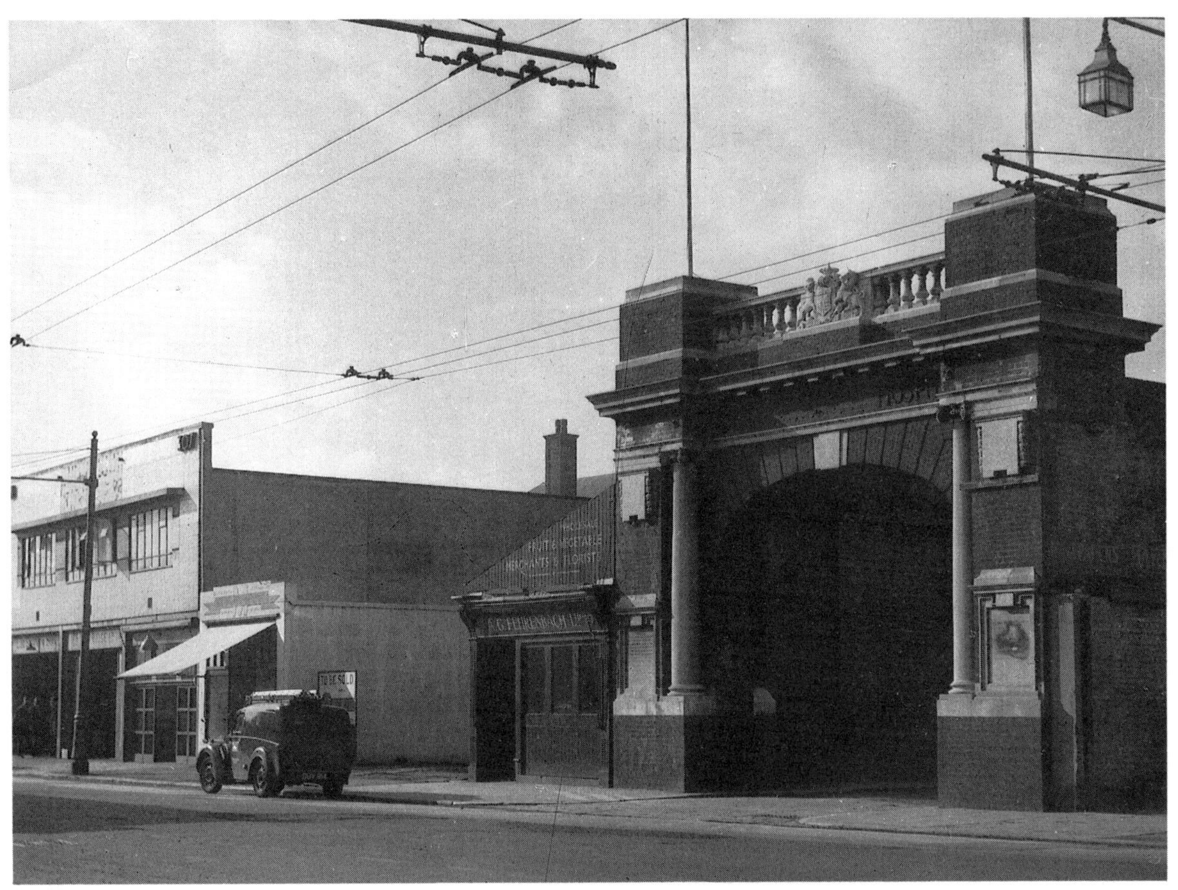

Memorial Gateway 1922.

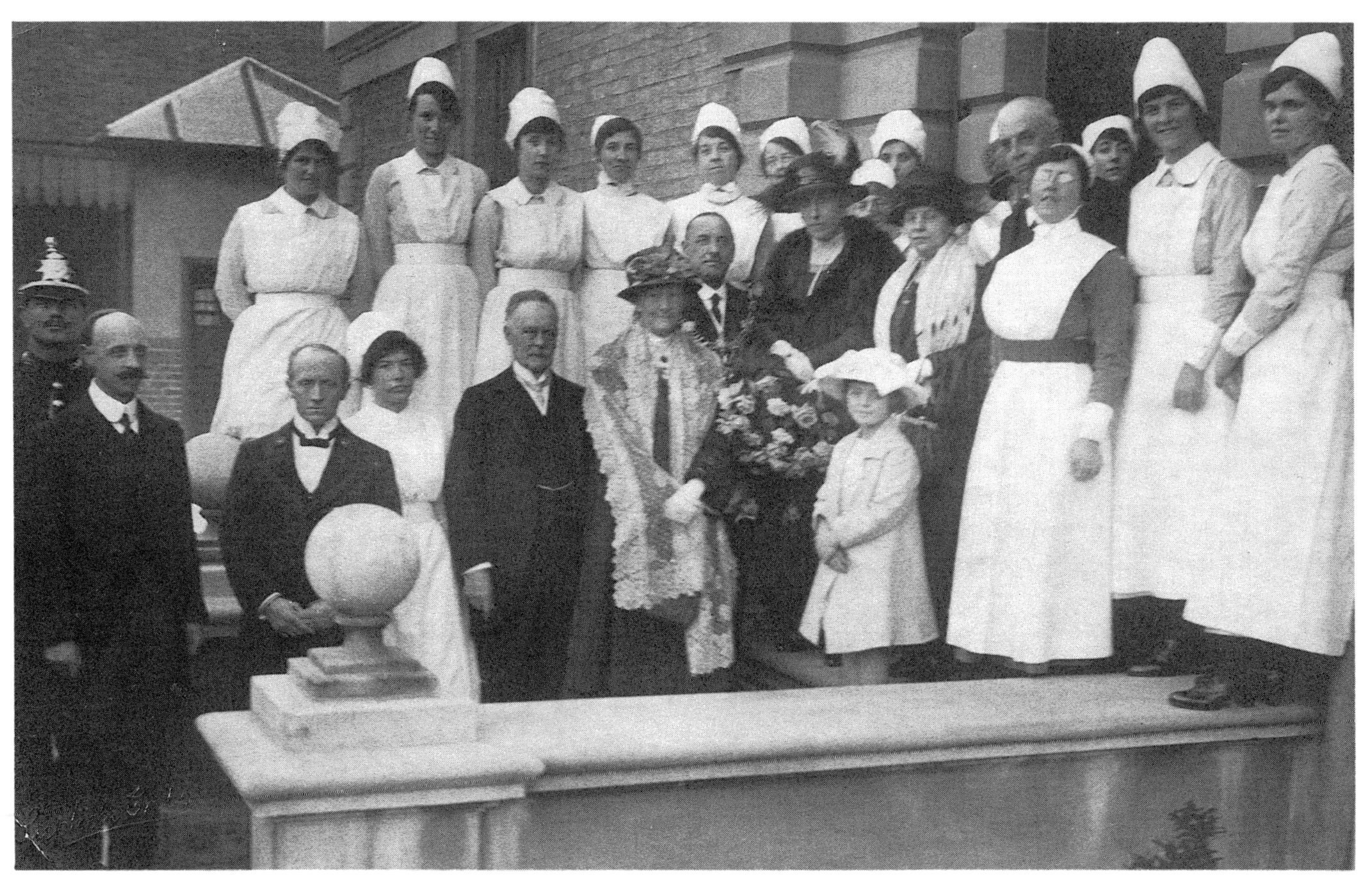

Group with the Princess, Sir Woolmer White, Alderman E. Porter and Mr Wagstaff, Hospital Secretary.

"A little Child shall lead them."
To commemorate the raising of £1000 for the endowment of two cots
by Mr F·G·Foster and Miss Doris Foster
Mayor and Mayoress of Portsmouth 1907-8

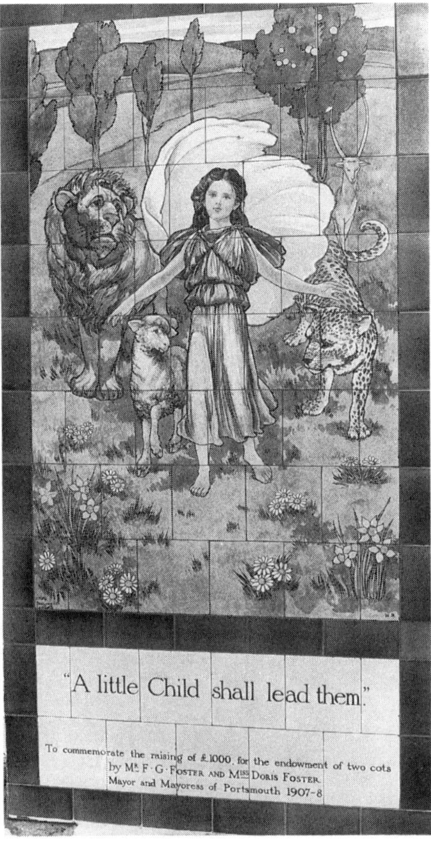

Wall Tiles, 1908.

Woolmer White, later Sir Woolmer White, a new out-patient department was opened, a far larger one than before and more in keeping with the increasing needs of the area.

The next priority was a better nurses home. To this end plans were drawn up by Mr C.W. Bevis and the contractor Mr G. Slater submitted a tender to build the home at a cost of £6,997. The building was opened on October 5th 1910 by Lady Curzon-Howe and it may have been the first memorial to King Edward VIII who had died on May 6th of that year. The nurses home overlooked the dockyard wall and was connected by a corridor to the old hospital buildings.

The Royal patronage was maintained when the new king, George V sanctioned the continuance of the prefix "Royal" to the name of the hospital.

In 1921 the Mayor, Sir John Timpson K.B.E. was raising money for the Portsmouth War Memorial Fund. From the fund he allocated £10,000 for improvements to the administration buildings and the rest to go to erect a Memorial Gateway. The site for this was made possible when Sir Woolmer White presented the hospital administrators with an old house which fronted Commercial Road. This was demolished and in its place was built the gateway so well remembered by all patients who ever attended either out-patients or the wards.

The opening ceremony was performed by H.R.H. Princess Victoria on May 19th 1922. The gateway was built of red brick and Portland Stone with the Royal Arms at the top of the archway. On one side of the upright at a suitable height was a receptacle built into the structure into which the general public could put silver paper which was then sold for funds. On the other a memorial stone on which was inscribed:

"This Gateway and extensive improvements to the hospital buildings form part of the Memorial raised by the inhabitants of Portsmouth to the memory of their fellow townsmen who gave their lives for their country in the Great War."

The opening ceremony as was usual with the Royal was a very well

Little Red Riding Hood.
Presented by the Staff and Students of the
Portsmouth Training College
as a
Souvenir of Miss E.L.White M.A.
Principal 1907-1932

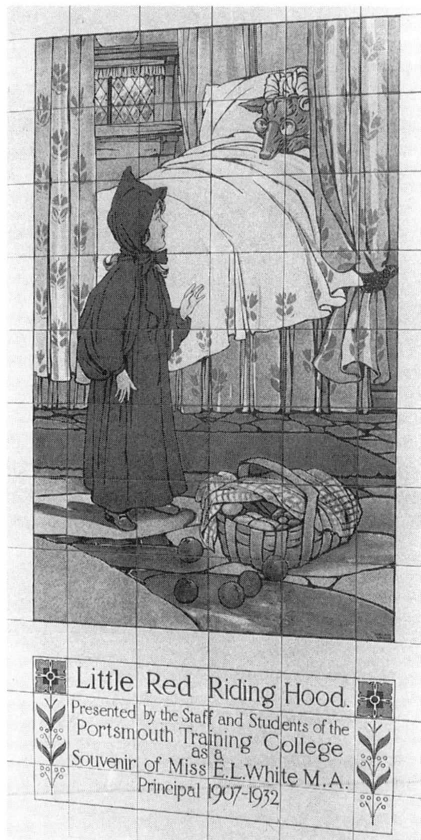

Wall Tiles, 1932.

attended affair. The people of Portsmouth turned out to watch and there was a large crowd in Commercial Road all ready to enjoy seeing the practical result of their fund raising. The Royal Irish Regiment provided both the band and the Guard of Honour.

Apart from the rearrangement of the administration block and the gateway, another extremely useful addition was a new corridor joining casualty to the wards. Also the corridor led to the kitchen which had been remolded when a grant from the Red Cross had made it possible.

So the memorial fund helped the hospital in more ways than one. It now had a direct entrance from Commercial Road, far more convenient for the new buildings than the ones in Fitzherbert Street had been.

On the occasion of the opening the Mayor was Alderman E Porter. In his speech he gave a brief history of the hospital showing how the royal connections had persisted since Prince Albert laid the foundation stone in 1847. He ended with a reference to the previous visit by Princess Helena Victoria when she opended the childrens ward in 1909. He also commented on her position as president of the Ladies Linen League. The whole day seemed to have passed in the usual style, another flag waving affair enjoyed by all. Very wisely, most of the great ceremonial occasions seemed to take place when good weather could at least be a possiblity.

The wards referred to in the speech were Young, Edward and Mary. Young was the children's ward and was named after Mr J.J. Young, chairman of the building committee and Mayor of Portsmouth in 1896. The second was the women's surgical and was named after the Prince and Princess of Wales.

In Young Ward there was a further tribute to the people of Portsmouth. Three murals made of Doulton tiles decorated the walls. They were six foot high and three foot wide, depicted biblical subjects and were affixed in 1908 ready for the opening. Later, in 1932, three more were added featuring nursery rhymes. They were in lovely bright colours and would have made the wards at least a little less frightening for small children.

Each panel had a dedication underneath and one is particularly interesting. It commemorates the raising of £1000 for the endowment of two cots by Mr G. Foster and Miss Doris Foster, Mayor and Mayoress of Portsmouth 1907/08. Mr Foster was a widower and Doris was his five year old daughter. By all accounts she was a highly successful Mayoress and took an active part in all suitable social functions. She may well have been the inspiration for the figure of the child in the picture entitled "A little child shall lead them."

These murals were fortunately saved and are still on display. Because of the interest of a few people they were saved and carefully restored by the craftsmen from the Jackfield Workshops in the Ironbridge Museum, Telford. The restoration took three years of work by these dedicated artists, but it was well worth the time and effort. They are now on show in a well lit position up the side of a staircase in the Portsmouth City Museum.

Another memorial which was almost completely lost when the hospital was demolished was the chapel. The windows were removed and they are still in store but the rest was destroyed. The Chapel was built as memorial to Sir Woolmer White and the money for it came from part of the £80,000 raised for the building of the final hospital block in 1930. This amount was raised largely through the efforts and generosity of Sir Woolmer who spent many years working for the good of the Royal.

The site was one which originally housed the museum built in memory of Mr Henry Rundle F.R.C.S. When his relatives were asked, they readily agreed that the building should be used. Until 1928 it had been used as a venue for the medical and surgical staff to hold meetings. Later it was a lecture room for the nurses; church services had been held there each week. Although a great deal of rebuilding would be necessary it was decided it was the obvious choice for the permanent chapel.

The roof was removed and a more suitable one replaced it; lancet windows were built in the walls and the sanctuary was added. An organ was presented by Sir Harold Pink and the stained glass windows were designed by Mr Lowson of the Faith Craft Studios, London.

The windows were donated by various people and revive memories of names long connected to the hospital; Alfred Grigsby, Henry Lapthorne, Sir Harold Pink, Henry Weston Burt, all members of the committee in one capacity or another plus Jane Read, founder of the Ladies Linen League, and from the medical staff were Mr T.A. Munro-Ford, surgeon, (this was donated by a grateful patient) and Dr Beverley-Steeds Bird, radiologist.

Anyone who worked in the X-ray departments of the town during and before the war will remember the two radiologists Dr Steeds-Bird and Dr R. Staley who worked tirelessly and always with consideration for both patients and staff.

The items in the sanctuary reminded those who saw them of past and present members of the nursing staff — Miss Alcock who left the hospital in 1921 and was once matron. Sister Bradbury was a sister of Edward and Mary Ward and who died in 1928; Miss Earle, once sister of Victoria Ward and later assistant matron; Sister Wellstead and Sister Dennis, also Miss Toogood, who was an X-ray department sister before the war. There are many people today who will have vivid memories of the Royal conjured up by the mention of these names.

The Chapel of St Barnabas was dedicated by Dr Neville-Lovett, first Bishop of Portsmouth, on April 30th 1936. The plaque showing the dedication read: "Praising God for the honoured memory of Woolmer White, Baronet, a munificient benefactor to the Hospital."

Unfortunately the chapel was extensively damaged in the last war. The windows had been removed for safe keeping but the rest needed extensive repairs. This was done in 1951 and on November 20th it was re-hallowed by Dr Lancelot Fleming, Bishop of Portsmouth.

1955 saw another change. The vestry was extended and was used as a rest room by relatives of dangerously ill patients. By 1958 it was realised that many more repairs and restorations were needed. The organ also needed replacing. By November 26th 1958 all the work was finished and the chapel was rededicated by the Right Reverend Bryan Robins, Assistant Bishop of Portsmouth.

There have been two references to the Linen League; this was one of the many ways in which the hospital funds were increased. It was started in 1911 and continued until the state took over in 1948. At that time £10,000 worth of linen was handed over. The ladies worked tirelessly to ensure that this very vital part of the hospital equipment was always available and in good order.

Another scheme to promote a reliable source of money apart from fund raising events (which were naturally one-off affairs) was the Home Saving Scheme. It was highly successful and simple to run. Those who joined in had to make a promise as follows — "I will place a box on the table every Sunday and invite those present to put in 1d. I will hand over to an authorised collector the amounts saved every three months." The first year saw five hundred and seventy-five taking part; by the second year the numbers had increased to nine hundred and forty.

Another lucrative idea was the Dockyard All-in Scheme. This was started in 1926 and both workers in the dockyard and in local businesses paid 2d per week, which entitled them and their families to hospital treatment. There was a fairly typical statement which said — "The scheme is naturally confined to the working classes." Today that sounds dreadful but it seemed to be taken for granted and did not appear to be resented. Although 2d sounds very little it brought in a useful sum at the end of the year at a time when unemployment was high and money tight.

In 1914 the Portsmouth *Evening News* started a fund to supply the hospital with Radium; £2,224 was subscribed and handed over to the hospital on the understanding that in no circumstances would it be removed and that it would be kept in safe custody. Also it must be made available to anyone in the area who needed it.

As early as 1906 a pathological department had been opened and in 1920 an X.ray Therapy machine was donated by Mrs Preston Jones. By 1923 Sir William Dupree had donated a portable X-ray set for use on the wards. In the main X-ray department that year 1,736 patients were X-rayed. It all points to a very busy institution where most facilities for giving maximum care were available.

Ten years later, in 1933, a completely new X-ray department was opened. It consisted of two rooms for diagnostic work and two joined by a control panel room for radio-therapy. Three changing cubicles, a staff room, reporting office, and dark room completed the unit. It occupied the area which was the male ward of the old hospital. Although a large part of the old building was destroyed during the war, the X-ray department was undamaged.

The last three wards to complete the original plan when the new hospital was started in 1899 were opened by Princess Patricia of Connaught in 1934.

The final building owed much to Sir Woolmer White who in 1929 pledged one pound for each pound raised in the appeal fund, up to £40,000. It not only spurred everyone on to greater efforts but also made the whole project seem more possible. When the block was opened it was dedicated as a memorial of thanksgiving for the recovery of King George V from a serious illness.

The wards were named Woolmer White, Lapthorne and Harold Pink. The second was after the chairman of the committee of the governing bodies 1925/35 and the third after the chairman of the management committee. Sir Harold Pink was also connected with the All-in Scheme from its inaugeration in 1926.

The same year the nurses home was extended and the casualty and pathological departments were enlarged. Another theatre was built in 1935 and dedicated to the memory of Mr C.P. Childs, senior surgeon for many years.

In 1941 the Royal suffered its first extensive damage. The casualty department was hit as well as the administration buildings and the matrons quarters. All the patients were safe but sadly there were casualties amongst the staff. One doctor, three nurses, two porters, one special constable and two naval men died. The Baring Block, which was built in 1868 was also destroyed.

In spite of quite a considerable loss of working area, the hospital managed to carry on until 1942 when things became impossible.

There was a heavy fire blitz and admissions were brisk but there were still empty beds. Mr Norman Lumb, the senior surgeon, came round the wards telling everyone that admission had to stop. The Sister was naturally shocked and said so in no uncertain terms. She was silenced by one short sentence. "I'm sorry Sister, the roof is burning."

The hospital had three hundred beds and accommodation for one hundred and nineteen nurses so the removal from the wards to the basement shelters was a great undertaking. This was achieved under the direction of Miss Keen and Miss Earle, the matron and assistant matron. All went smoothly but when the in-patients were re-admittted to St James' it was with a feeling of relief. That hospital did have some damage but it was mainly confined to the grounds; also it was in a far less vulnerable position. The nearness of the Dockyard to the Royal almost made it a legitimate target.

The out-patients department remained in Commercial Road and so did the X-ray unit. A portable set was kept at St James' for in-patients and some out-patients. The radiographers worked a rota system, one working at St James' a week at a time. There had to be twenty-four hour cover and this was arranged by one radiographer being on duty and stand by duty for twenty-four hours once a week, plus one complete week-end in rotation. This worked well unless there were air raid casualties who needed urgent attention. Mr Paul Murray, the surgical registrar, thought it best to let them recover from shock unless his examination found the need for urgent diagnostic X-rays. So only essential work was done after hours. An exception had to be made when a convoy of men from the battle-fields came in during the night. They had to be ready to be discharged as soon as possible the next day. The beds had to be ready for the next emergency as soon as the

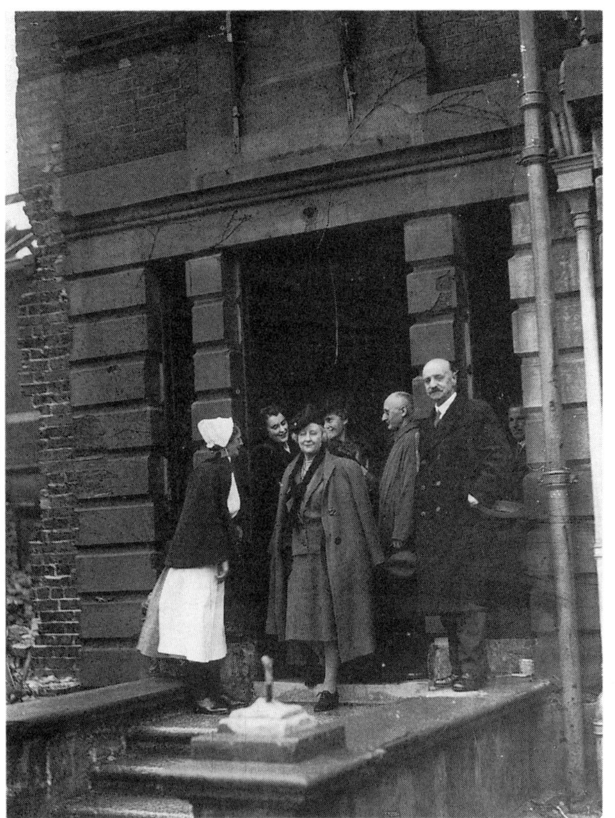

Assistant Matron, Miss Earle and Mr Wagstaff on the steps of the bombed administration buildings.

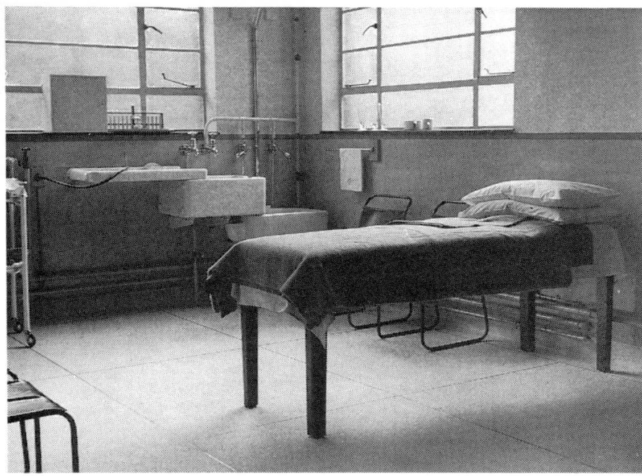

Corner of Out-patients.

patients could be sent to their permanent hospitals. In this case it was decided that the disturbance caused was justified.

The war did not stop social life, and parties at Christmas still went on. The surgeons carried on the tradition of carving the bird at all the special dinners on the wards. The nurses had their Christmas dinner and the domestics theirs. The domestics were waited on by the nurses at table, they also did the washing up afterwards. Naturally the wards were decorated and carols were sung.

The care of the nurses was in the hands of the Home Sister, Sister Harvey and the Medical Superintendent Dr Farncombe. The best was got out of the food available. Potatoes were usually baked in their jackets to preserve vitamins. Carrots were served in many guises one being a sort of pudding no doubt excellent but far from tempting when seen on the plate. There were vitamin tablets on the table at each meal. The standard of health seemed very good, at least as far as can be remembered.

One of the constant troubles at the Royal where the dining room was in the old building was mice. Any member of staff who, because of an emergency had to work through supper time had her meal saved. That meant so often sitting alone in a big empty room. Or at least empty of humans. The only way to survive was to sit on one chair with feet firmly planted on another whilst mice ran back and forth across the floor in their hundreds.

The mice were indestructable; cats did their best but there were plenty more mice to replace any which were caught. The area had been badly bombed and no doubt mice can be bombed out like humans so there was a constant supply for the duration. For some reason they did not seem to have any adverse effect on the health of either the patients or staff.

During their stay at St James', the staff lived at Foster Hall at the end of Locksway Road, so the mice infestation did not destroy the peace of the meals there. The stay at St James' was a fairly short one. As soon as the bombing diminished in 1943, the wards reopened at the Royal.

In 1945 Miss Keen O.B.E. retired as matron, a post she had held since 1921. She was no stranger to casualty work for she had volunteered to go to Greece in 1913 to nurse the wounded at the time of the Balkan War. She worked in Salonika for several months and described it as an interesting experience but some of the patients gave a lot of trouble; they were sure they were far too ill to be washed. She accepted the award of the O.B.E. in January 1943 as official recognition of the work done by the entire nursing staff. On February 15th 1946, Miss Earle the assistant matron also retired. They were two very remarkable ladies. It is a happy thought that Miss Keen's name has survived the final closure of the Royal. There is a ward named after her at Queen Alexandra Hospital, Cosham.

Gradually the hospital was rebuilt. An enlarged X-ray department was opened in 1949 and the next year the pathological laboratory was constructed. The orthopaedic and fracture clinics were built on the

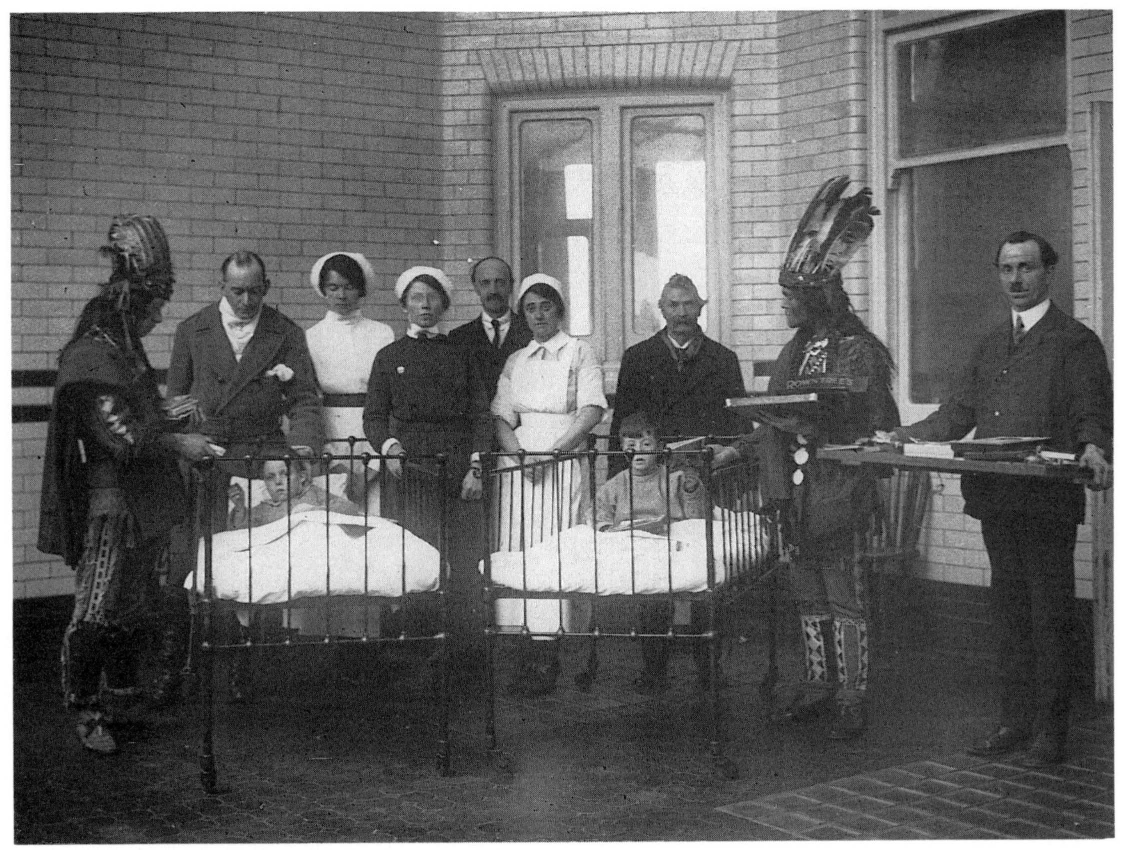

Miss Keen, Matron with Mr Wagstaff giving presents in the children's ward.

site previously occupied by the bombed casualty department. These were opened by H.R.H. Princess Alice Duchess of Gloucester in 1952. The combined clinics were named Gloucester Ward in honour of the occasion.

Building still continued and in 1952 the Lord Mayor Alderman Johnson opened the new accident and emergency department. The department of physical medicine is always an important part of any orthopaedic and accident hospital. As the Royal was the main accident centre for the whole city, it was essential the facilities were adequate. The rebuilding of the department was started and it was finally rehoused in the new building in 1950. A gymnasium was also a necessary part of rehabilitation and one was opened in 1957. Also in that year Princess Alexandra of Kent opened the new out-patients department. There was another Royal visit earlier when Princess Margaret toured the hospital in 1952. So the fifties were a very important decade in the Royal's history when much of the damage caused during the war was restored.

Still work went on, a new dental and orthopaedic department was built, a very necessary service for an accident hospital, as injuries to jaw and teeth were becoming more common in road accidents. The unit was opened by the then Minister of Health, Mr Enoch Powell M.P.

These alterations and repairs did not always go smoothly. The pathological department was built only after an initial application was turned down. A re-application to the Ministry of Health in September 1946, two months after the first one, achieved the desired result. Even so it was three years later before it finally opened. For five years casualties were attended to in a temporary Nissen hut. The easing of the bed situation was more immediate.

After the war twenty-six beds were at once made available for the Royal patients at St Mary's and one month later, in December 1946, Queen Alexandra's helped to bridge the gap. The next year York Ward was completely renovated and opened as a woman's medical ward.

Money was still being donated over and above the amount officially

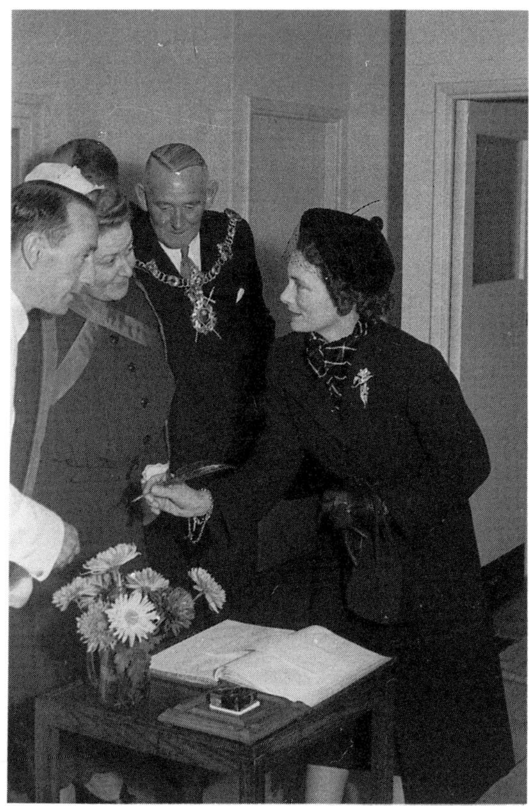

The Duchess of Gloucester, Matron De La Court and Sir Denis Daley, Mayor.

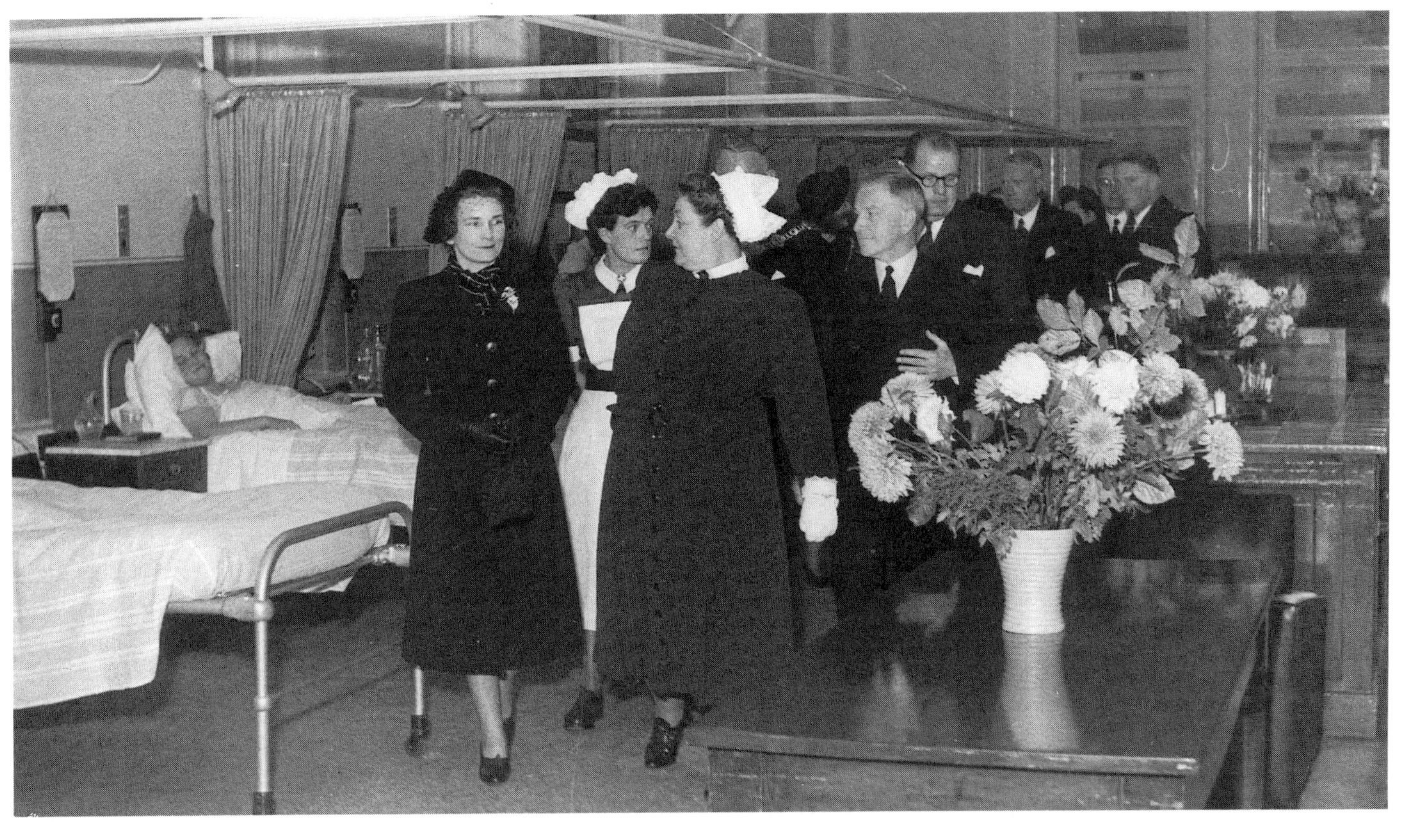

Touring the wards with Sister Winter and Senior Surgeon Mr Hillman.

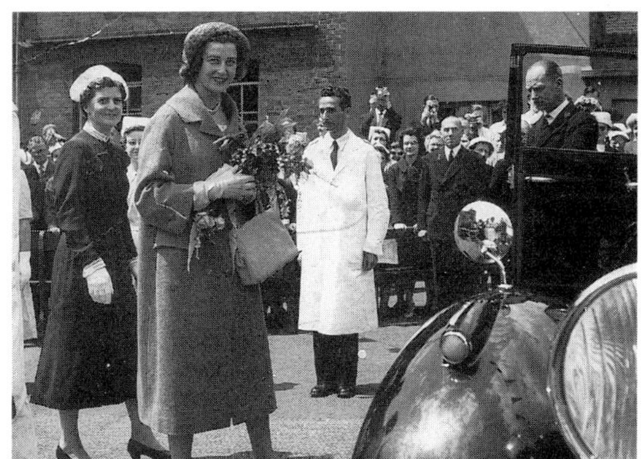

Princess Alexandra with Matron Ashton and head porter Mr Pottinger.

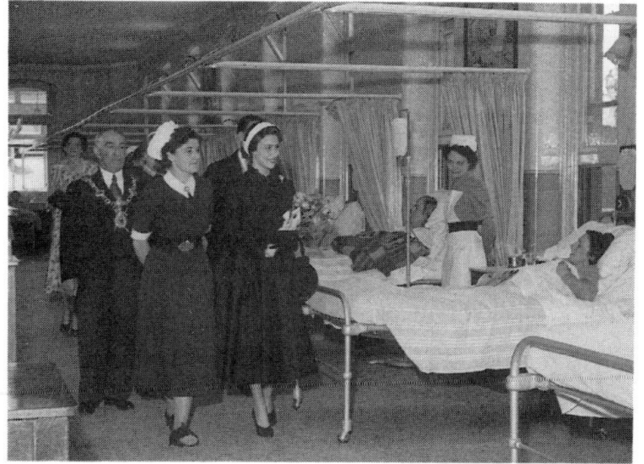

Edward and Mary Ward with Princess Margaret, Sister Aldridge and Alderman J. Johnson. 1952.

allocated by the authorities as war damage payments. Just before the war an anonymous donor had given £1000 to be spent on the X-ray department. After the war, funds were being raised to endow a cot in memory of Dr Farncombe who had been medical superintendent during the war. The Lord Mayor's Fund aimed at raising £15,000 towards general necessities for the Royal. On the list of subscribers was the name of a South African lady, so help was not just coming from local people. The good will was still there but it was an uphill task as the damage had been considerable.

One great source of controversy was the decision to demolish the Memorial Gateway in 1958. Owing to the bombing and the resultant reorganisation of the buildings around it, the gate was no longer considered safe. The readers of the Portsmouth *Evening News* had other ideas and a brisk correspondence in the letters column ensued. The authorities won in the end but whether they were right is debatable. The gate had been well built of pre-stressed concrete and proved extremely difficult to demolish. It had withstood two land mines which had come down in the forecourt without moving an inch. But it had to go and perhaps it marked the beginning of the end of the Royal. Twenty years later, the days of the hospital were numbered. It was only because of delays in building the new general hospital on Portsdown hill that the end did not come sooner.

But still improvements went on in both large and small ways. The League of Friends worked tirelessly for the good of the patients. In 1959 £417 was raised by a special effort and two Ripple beds were bought which added greatly to the comfort of long stay and very ill patients.

In June 1962 it was decided that Woolmer White ward would be turned into a private wing. This did not last long as nine years later pay beds was phased out and the ward reverted to its normal use. Even as late as 1962 improvements continued and a new day room was opened in September of that year.

But it was a losing battle. Too much needed to be done and the ideas

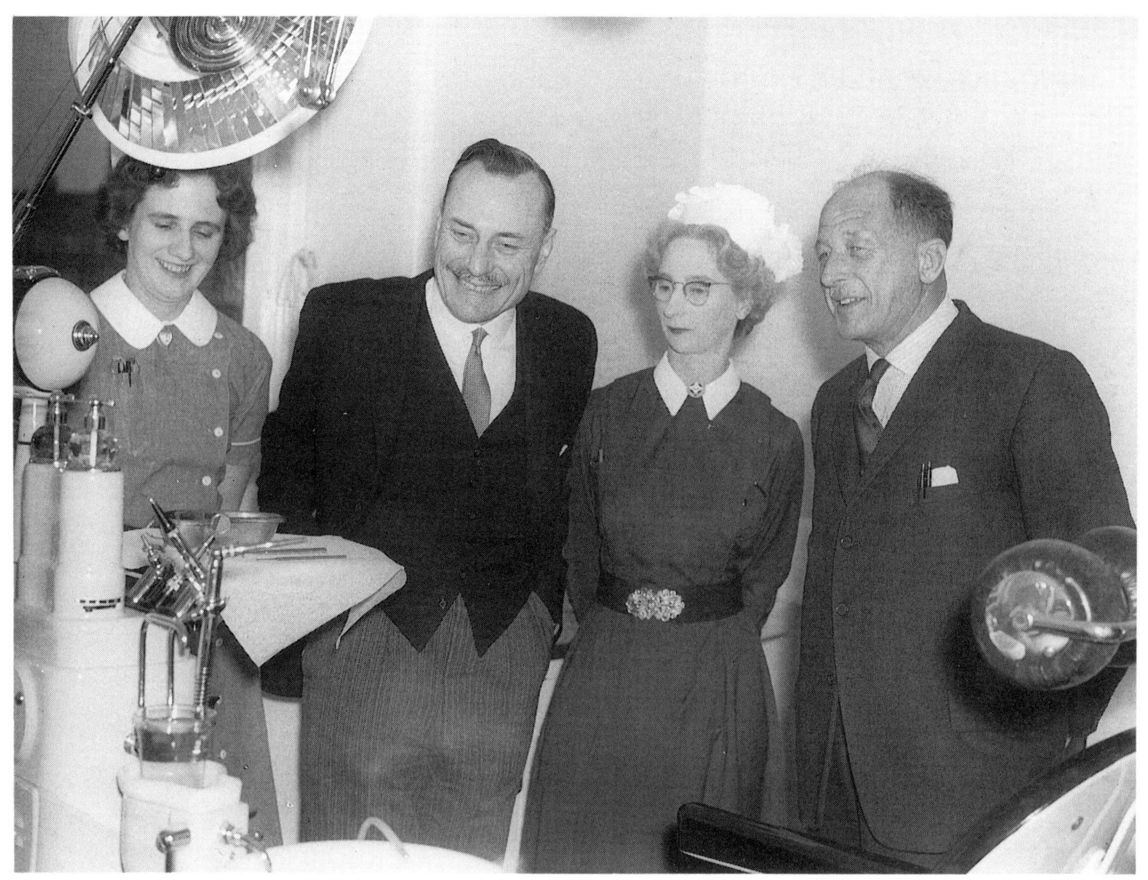

Opening of the new Dental Department by Mr Enoch Powell M.P. then M.O.H.

of the Health Service were much in favour of large regional hospitals where comprehensive facilities were available under one roof. Also, with increased traffic in the centre of the town, having a hospital in Commercial Road was no longer sensible. Rushing emergencies through was becoming a nightmare and there was no available space on which to expand. Car parking, the great problem of this cluttered age, was impossible.

On January 1st 1978, the last Christmas party before the hospital was due to be closed was held. In March the following year, the League of Friends had their last meeting. By May only two patients remained. When they were finally transferred to Queen Alexandra shortly afterwards the long history of the Royal Portsmouth Hospital ended.

By April 1984 the bulldozers had started their work and were fulfilling a six-month contract to clear the site which initially was intended for office blocks, a petrol station, a D.I.Y. store. Like most hospitals, the Royal had its ghost. She was said to appear on York Ward though some were equally convinced that her area of haunting was the Harold Pink Ward. No doubt any self-respecting ghost could manage both at once. But what happens to ghosts when they are evicted?

The next large hospital to have been opened after the Royal was the Borough of Portsmouth Lunatic Asylum. It was renamed later but that was its title to begin with. Seventy-five acres of land was brought at the cost of £14,000 for the building of a hospital initially intended to house four hundred and ten patients. It was situated between Velder Creek and Eastney Lake, on rough and uncultivated land, a deliberate decision as the care of the grounds by the patients would be part of their treatment. The aim being always to reinstate them in society as soon as possible.

The plans were drawn up by the Portsea architect Mr George Rake; the foundation stone was laid by the Mayor William Pink on July 11th 1876. After some unforseen delays, the hospital was opened by Mayor W. King on September 30th 1879. A lavish lunch followed the ceremony attended by Prince Edward Saxeweimer and many distinguished guests. Judging by the editorial of the *Hampshire Telegraph* this was met with fairly widespread disapproval. It read as follows:

> "There seems to be something incongrous at first sight in the festive celebration of the opening of a new lunatic Asylum. A solemn service or perhaps no service at all, would appear more in harmony with the event, and with the view of the majority of the people with regard to it. But the ordinary Englishman is so wedded to routine, and has been brought up in the belief that no public ceremony is complete which does not include a deal of eating and drinking."

Patients were arriving by the middle of October although building was still going on. It was three months before the farm buildings, the chapel and the boundary wall had been completed. By this time over four hundred patients had been admitted.

As well as the selection of the site with land for cultivation the whole design of the hospital was aimed at rehabilitation. The idea was to be as self supporting as possible.

By the time the buildings were completed there were workshops for tailoring, shoemaking, brewing, carpentry and laundry work. Gardeners and farmworkers were well catered for, as were bakers and general cooks. There was always plenty of work for sewing women of all grades of ability.

The total cost of all the buildings was £120,000. By December 31st 1880, four hundred and fifty-three patients had been admitted.

The wage received by the heads of departments varied considerably. The farm baliff with house, garden produce and free milk earned £54 per annum, whilst the baker with lodgings, rations and washing free had a great deal less, £15 per annum.

When their physical and mental condition permitted there was never any difficulty in finding suitable people with the necessary qualifications to do the work in the hospital grounds and in the hospital. A list of occupations was made on admission in 1885 and a selection from the thirty different activities reads as follows-

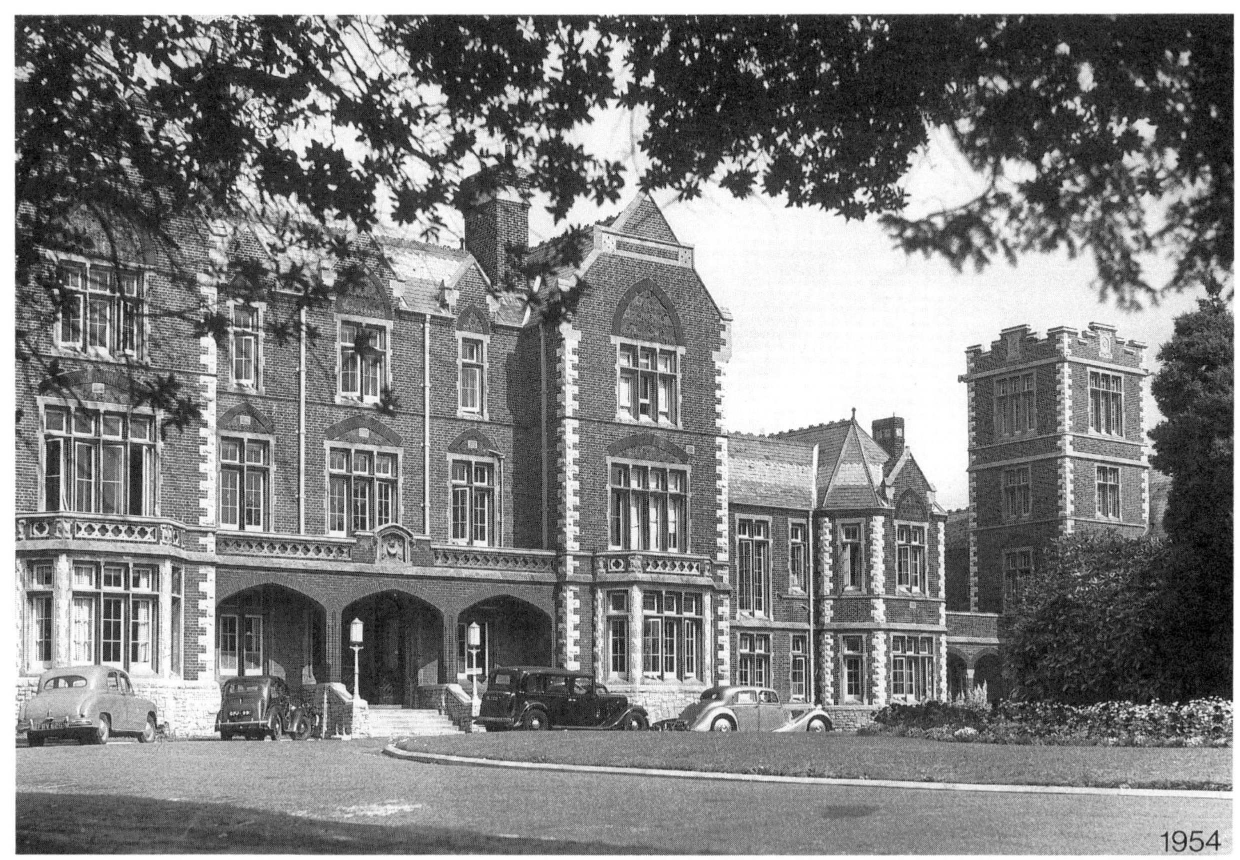

St James Hospital, Milton.

Artist, baker, bricklayer, butcher, boot-maker, tailor, stockman, and amongst the more unusual skills, or at least the present day, sword-maker, horse-clipper, French polisher and coal porter. There was also a clerk in holy orders and a stockbroker.

The women had a less varied list with fifteen different types of domestic work but there was also a little variation with a prison matron, a stay worker and an eating house keeper.

The reasons for their illness were also noted. Apart from mental disease, there were jealousy, overwork, anxiety, domestic trouble, poverty, fright, religion, excitement and disappointment in love. And right at the end — no known cause. It all sounds very familiar and perhaps little has changed in the last hundred years.

The rules governing the conduct of the nurses were clearly defined.

Leave once a fortnight from 2 p.m. - 9.45 p.m. and every second Sunday 4 p.m. - 9.45 p.m. After twelve months of good behaviour, one week's holiday. After two years, ten days to be divided as the medical superintendent wished. No smoking in the bedrooms or on duty and should a patient escape through the negligence of the staff, the nurse concerned would have to pay for the expense incurred to get him or her back. As the scale of pay for nurses was decidedly low no doubt the thought of money involved would have helped to increase vigilance. A male attendant in charge received £40 per annum and a female only had £32. A male second class had £20 and a female second class £16.

Fines were also imposed for misconduct or negligence. All staff were required to sign a paper promising never to gossip about the patients or the affairs of the asylum. They also acknowledged the right of the committee of visitors and the medical superintendent to discharge them without notice for intemperance of disobedience.

The medical superintendent was also subjected to strict rules. He had to be a legally qualified physician or surgeon. Although he was the chief officer of the asylum and was allowed no duties outside the hospital, he was completely ruled by the authority of the committee.

There were two committees. One, the committee of visitors was formed by members of the town council headed by the Mayor; two of its members were auditors. This group had overall authority and orders, other than the day-to-day costs, all had to have their signatures.

The other, the house of management committee met twice a month. They were responsible for the day-to-day running of the institution, wages, stores, and the condition of the kitchens and the wards; in fact all those items which needed constant supervision.

Although Portsmouth Council were responsible for the building of the hospital, they were answerable to the principle secretary of State at Whitehall. So the welfare of the patients was ensured at several levels.

The patients were admitted from a considerable area, from London, Brighton and Reigate, even as far as Windsor; and a few were recommended by the Prison Commissioners. Amongst the four hundred and fifty listed in 1880 were sixteen private patients. So even a century ago there were paying patients in general hospitals.

A further fourteen acres of land were bought in 1893 and a sanatorium was built for the care of infectious cases. But this did little to relieve the overcrowding which throughout its history has plagued St James'.

There have always been great efforts made to try to keep the problem under control but it sometimes must have seemed impossible. In an attempt to improve things, as more hospitals were opened in other parts of the country for mental treatment, patients from those areas were discharged to be nearer home. This naturally pleased both patient and relations; the latter often complained that they could not afford to travel such long distances to visit.

As this was happening, work was going ahead in St James' itself. Four Villas — King, Pink, Brunel and Dickens — were opened. Today, Brunel is partly used as a self-contained flat for six people so that patients can look after themselves in a sheltered environment before moving out to a house in the town. There they will still be under the care of the community services but will be responsible for the day-to-day running of their lives.

Right from the start, rehabilitation has been the aim. To this end, reading was encouraged. The problem was where to keep the books. In 1897 there was some difficulty when it was found they were being kept in the medicine cupboard, which was naturally locked. Then it was found that the library consisted of six bibles, one prayer book and two hymn books, hardly a wide choice. The chaplain was responsible for the reading matter so it was suggested he should do something about it.

And something was done very quickly. To celebrate the Queen's jubilee, one hundred books were given by the library committee and newspapers were donated by local people.

The problem of caring for the books persisted. Even as late as 1933 the controversy about locked cupboards still went on. By that date, the books had graduated from the medicine to the document files. Naturally they were still locked. The staff were responsible for their safe keeping and felt that if they were freely available some patients would make short work of them. In spite of their possible distruction it was decided they would be put in a place accessable to all.

Two years later it appears the risk was worth taking. It was noted by the committee when they made their rounds that patients were all enjoying the books and periodicals available in the wards. The concern about reading matter still went on and in 1953 it was agreed a part-time librarian would be engaged to make the whole arrangement more efficient. A long way from the resident clergyman and his bible in the medicine cupboard.

One of the jobs of the committee was to curb any tendency to overspend. When it was recommended a piano should be bought they made it quite clear that it should be secondhand. At the same time the idea of musical boxes for the less able patients was put forward. A small amount of money was allocated to buy pictures and prints to brighten up the walls.

The musical box idea came to nothing but the pianos did materialise. A year later in 1886 all the female wards had pianos and the male wards had both a bagatelle and a billiard table each. Outdoor entertainment varied; to celebrate Queen Victoria's Jubilee there were sports and a special tea on the lawn. Naturally this was a one-off treat, but picnics did take place every year. For this annual event a venue some distance away was always chosen. For people so rarely outside the grounds, the journey must have been as great a treat as the picnic itself. One day they would go to Uppark near Harting on another to South Farm, Forestside. As between three and four hundred went each time, it must have needed a great deal of organisation by the staff.

The record of the cricket team seemed good too, though there is no mention of the names of the opponent teams. In 1894 they had played twenty-five matches and won seventeen. Also at the time a reed band was formed to play out doors and a quadrill band to play for dances.

When electricity was installed in 1896 at a cost of £554.4s 7d (an extraordinary figure if only for its accuracy) the difference it made to both patients and staff must have been considerable. It was nineteen years later when a film projector was put up in the recreation hall and another twenty, in 1933, when talkies came to St James'. Twenty years after that, television sets were provided for all the wards. By this time there were weekly cinema performances and dances. There were also frequent concerts, some given by the council for music in hospitals.

Trips to the Coliseum, the Empire Theatre and the Theatre Royal were arranged from time to time so the patients were able to extend their experience of living outside the walls.

Until a fully trained occupational therapist was employed in 1964 this side of the patients treatment was supervised by the nurses. It was so successful that long stay patients were able to get outside contracts and the resultant profits were given to the workers.

Because the hospital was largely self-supporting, the charge on the

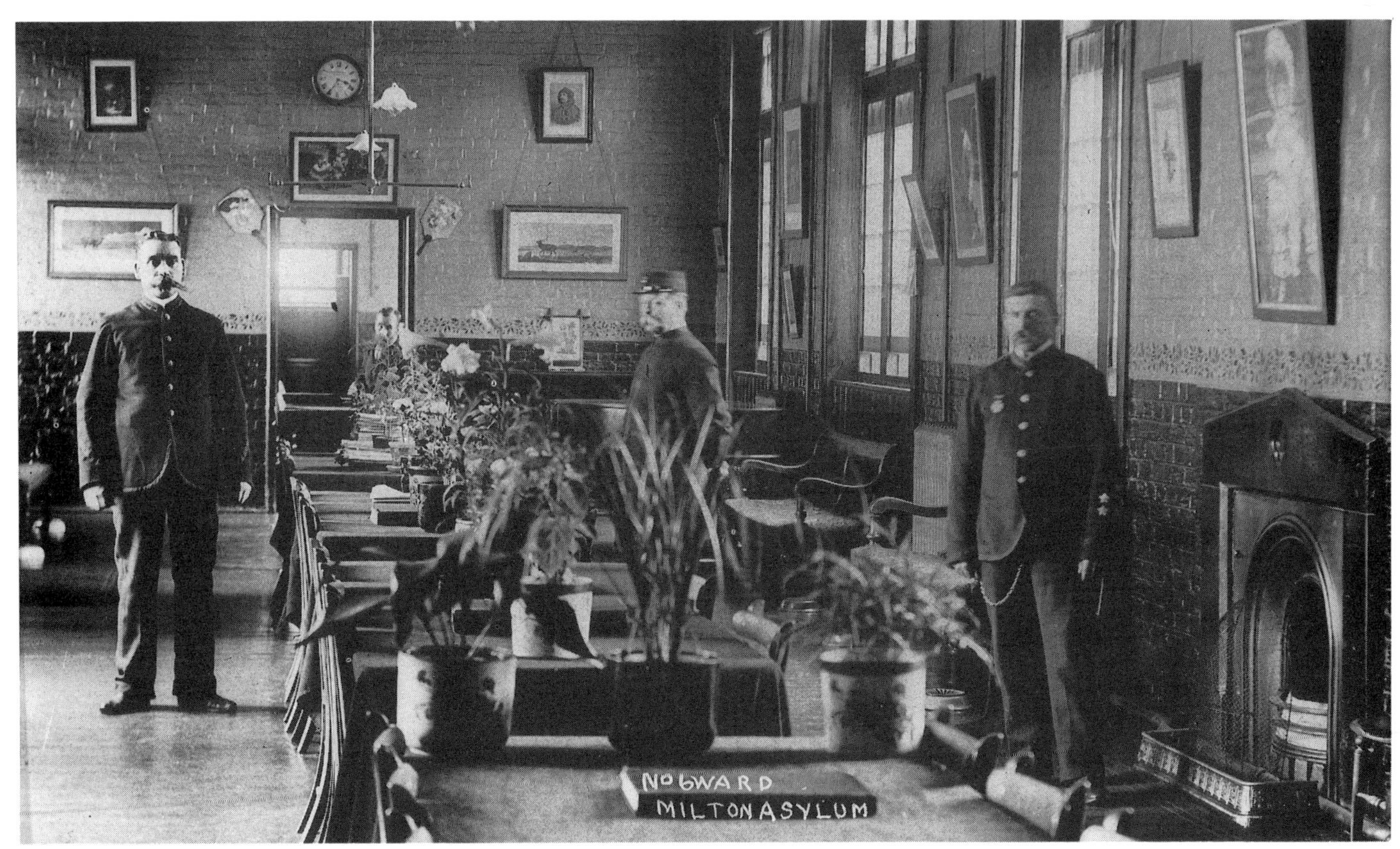

Mens Ward. With books and pictures.

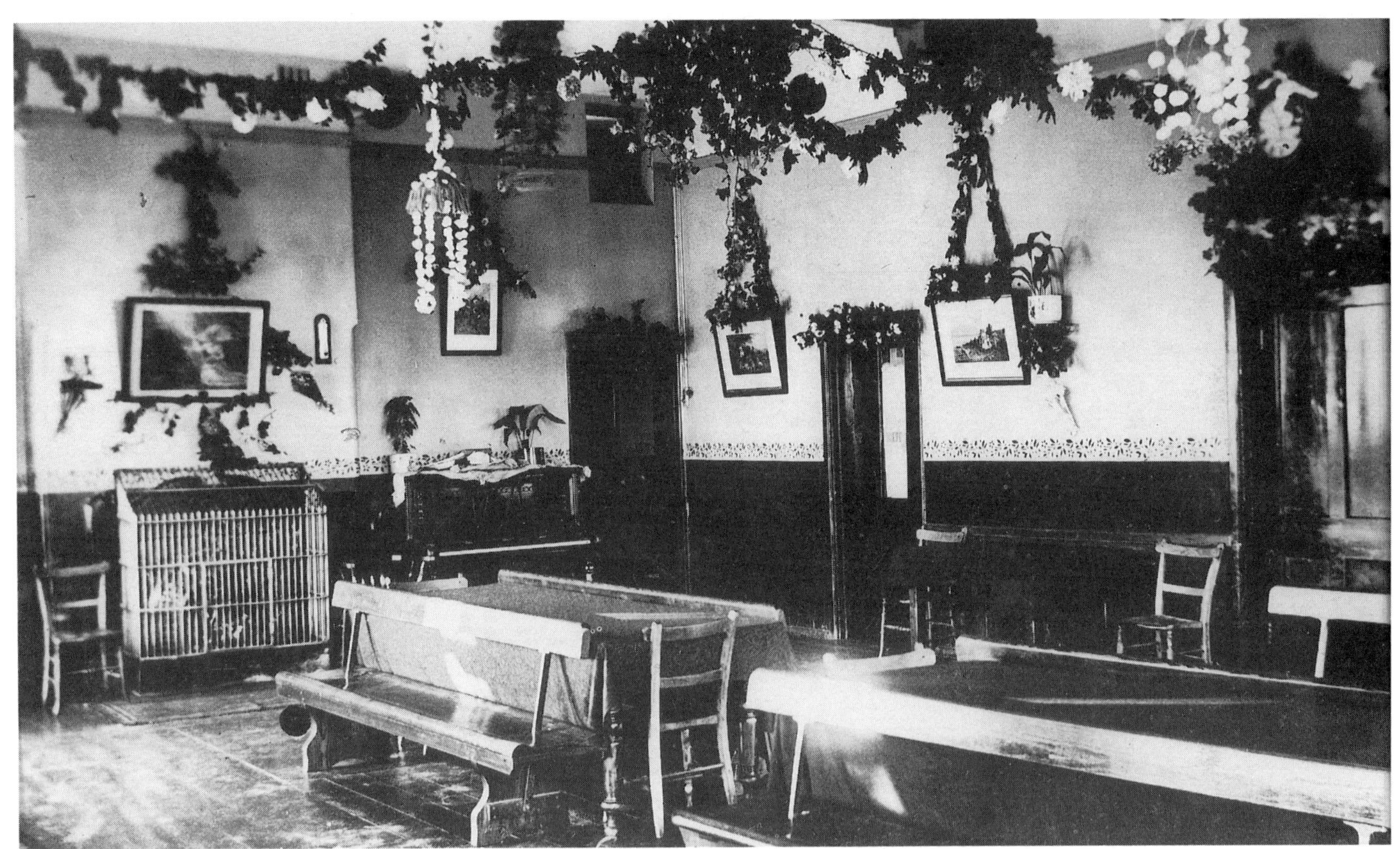

Ward decorated for Christmas showing one of the pianos.

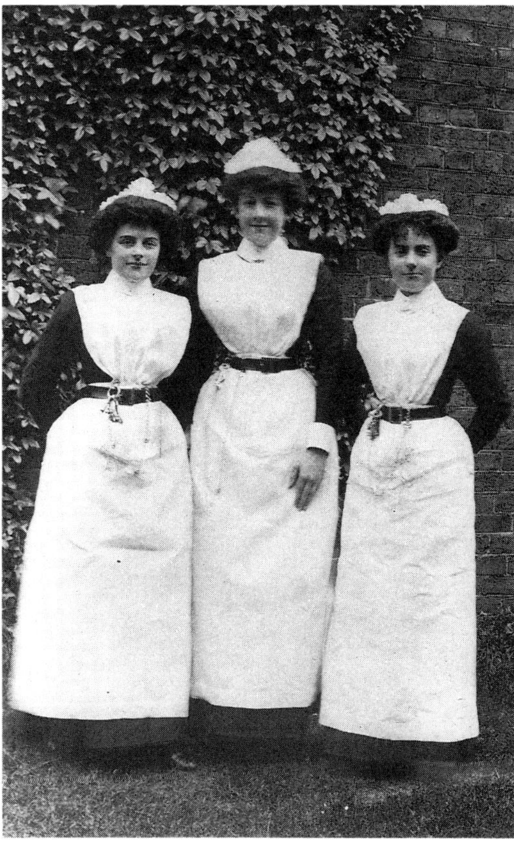

Nurses with ward keys on belt.

borough for each patient was not great. In 1880, 13s 1d was the cost of feeding and caring for the local patient. There was a slight increase to 14d for patients from other districts. Private patients were charged 16s — £1. These costs varied from time to time according to the availablitiy of farm produce. In 1883 the cost was reduced to 11s 1d saving the borough £2,500 over the year.

The farm was a profitable undertaking. In 1898 the stock consisted of three horses, fourteen cows, four heifers, three calves and eighty-seven chicken. To this list, pigs were added later. In 1914 profits from the farm and gardens amounted to £201. 6s 10½ by the next year it showed a further increase and the sum was £729. 18.10. When the Americans took over St James' for a short while at the end of the Great War using the farmland and gardens to erect hutments, they handed over £1,455 1s as compensation for the loss of crops. The extremely exact bookwork with calculations to literally the last penny seemed to be the practice of that time.

In 1965 the farm was finally closed down. One hundred and sixty acres had already been sold leaving sixty still under cultivation. So the last farm on Portsea Island was no more. It was rather sad as it was still a profitable insitution both financially and for the treatment point of view. In one year it had supplied pork, fruit and vegetables to the value of £5,056 to the hospital and £3,760 to other institutions in the area.

War did not affect St James' in the same way as it did the casualty and general hospitals but in some ways it was equally disturbing. During the Boer War six reservists were called up. At that time there were only thirty-nine male nurses so that number must have caused a real shortage of staff. The number of patients was constantly increasing, the original four hundred and ten was only an ideal figure, the real one was nearly half that again. Eventually, in spite of all the efforts to keep the numbers down, there were over one thousand patients in St James'. By that time there had been a lot of extra building.

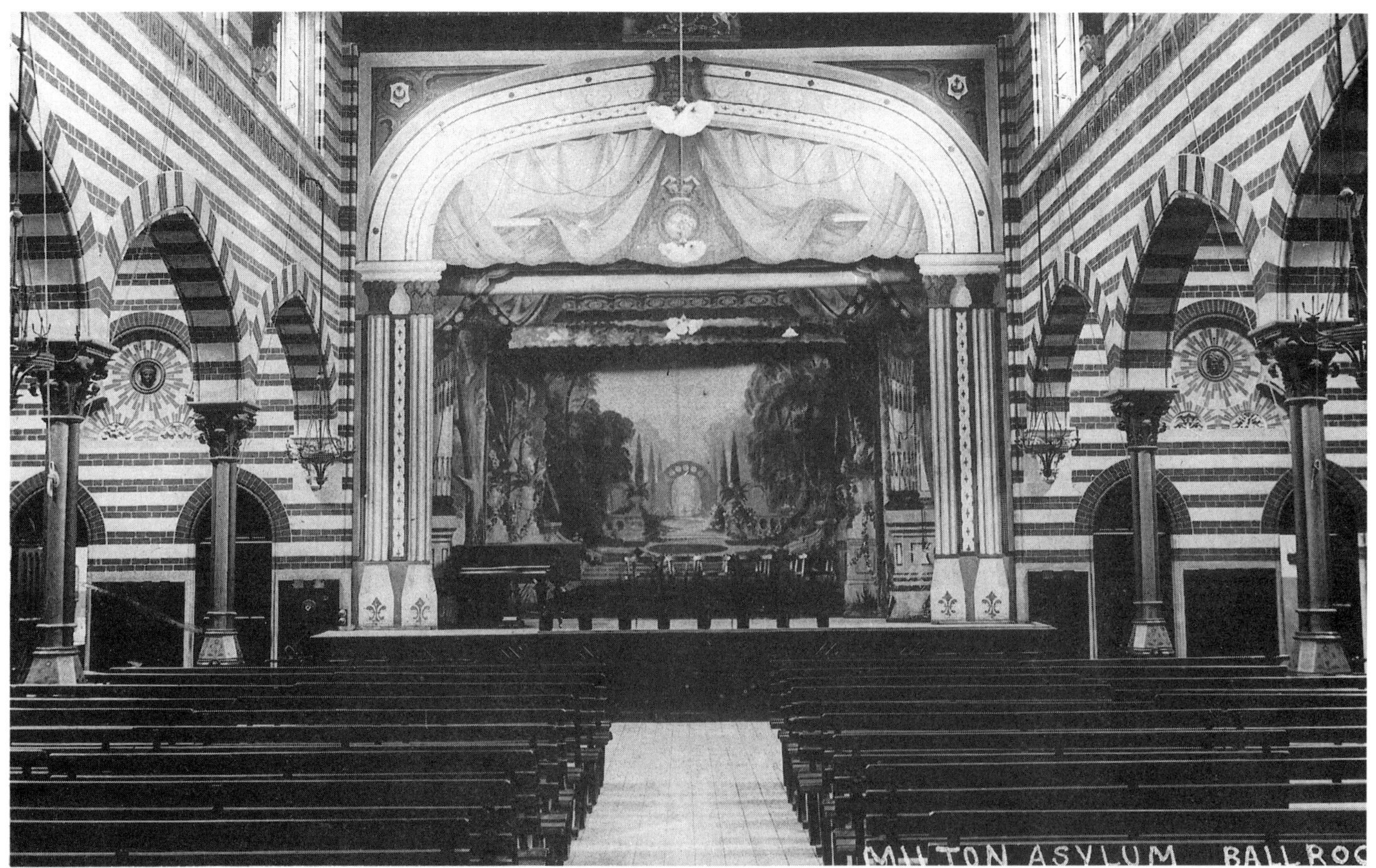

The Ball Room.

The families of enlisted men were cared for by the hospital and an allowance of seven shillings a week was paid to the wives of the men who were away. At the end of the 1914-1918 war, disruption was complete. As had already been mentioned the whole hospital was taken over by the Americans and became the U.S.A. Base Hospital 33. The evacuation of the mental patients went smoothly. They went to various other institutions in the country; the ambulances covered 3,604 miles during the operation.

The hospital was transformed into a completely equipped general unit with three operating theatres, pathological department, X-ray opthalmic, ear nose and throat and dental departments. The staff came with them and they specialised in all brances of surgery.

Twelve hutments were built in the grounds and every available bed was needed. As well as the wounded, one boat load of influenza cases was landed in Southampton. They were all admitted to St James'. The influenza epidemic was dangerous and widespread and is still remembered by the generation who experienced it. Tents were erected for the less ill.

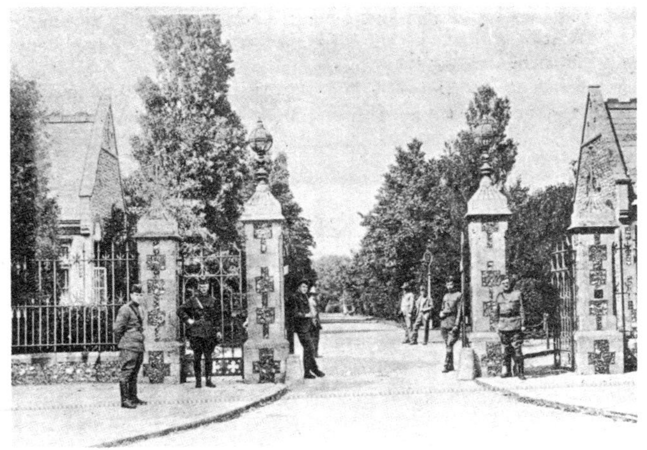

Hospital Gates during the American occupation, 1918.

Although the occupation was short, from July 22nd 1918 until early in February 1919, 3,000 patients were treated during that time.

In the last war, once more wards were handed over for the treatment of casualties. This time it was the Royal Hospital which needed help and one hundred and twenty beds were made available. Thirty were kept for routine medical and surgical cases and the rest for air raid victims. Later it was a short stay unit for army wounded. The wards were staffed by Royal nurses and medical staff, the nurses being accommodated in the students home at Foster Hall, Locksway Road.

This was the position for two years until the Royal was re-opened in Commercial Road and the wards could again be used for their original purpose.

Fourteen years after the hospital was first opened, it was decided that the nursing staff should have instruction in first aid and nursing. Today it seems impossible that such a difficult and specialised field of nursing could be in the hands of completely untrained people.

Three years later, lectures were being given in conjunction with the Medico-Phychological Society. The following year there were nine successful candidates who sat the exam set by the society. Each was given a badge and a prize of £1.

By the early 1930s, a high proportion of the staff were either registered or had passed their preliminary exams. By 1948 the nurses were spending two months at St Mary's to get general nursing experience before returning to complete their training. By 1960, quite a high proportion of the staff were state-registered nurses as well as registered mental nurses. In 1975, the method of examination was changed. Instead of a national basis for assessment, each training school became responsible for training and examining their own nurses.

When it was first opened, St James' was called the Borough of

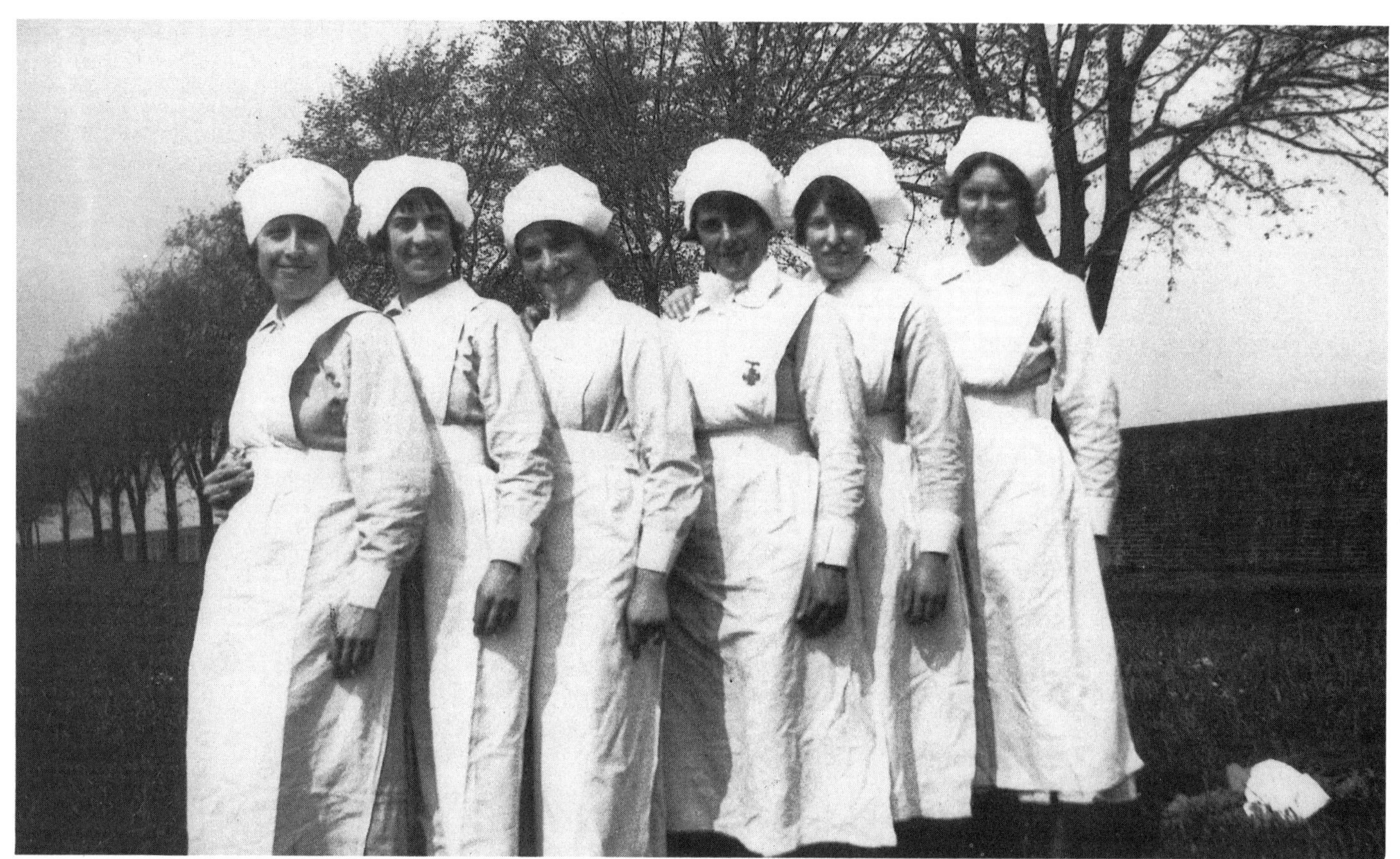

Nurses with staff nurse showing her hospital badge.

Portsmouth Lunatic Asylum. This was changed to the Portsmouth Borough Mental Hospital in 1920. When this was changed to St James' Hospital for Nervous and Mental Diseases, times were really getting more enlightened. But that was not until 1937. In 1960 the name was changed again and it became St James' Psychiatric Hospital.

As the name altered so did the way of referring to mental illness. In Victorian days there was little regard for the feelings of the mental patient and his or her relations. It was not considered wrong to refer to them as luncatics and paupers. In 1910 there was a note made by the committee saying that idiot boys should not be housed in the adult wards. So at least that was a step in the right direction even if it did not go nearly far enough.

When the villas were first opened, there was an entry which said they would benefit both private patients and paupers. The private patients, also called gentlemen, paid a guinea and a half per week. It was said: "This allowed a more delicate diet than was possible in the main building and they were comfortable in their new quarters." In spite of the delicate diet, their presence in the institution was justified by a profit gained for the borough of £2,231 4s up to March 1910.

Perhaps the Great War gave a greater awareness of the need to break down social barriers. Whatever the cause, the result was good. In 1918 it was admitted the term pauper used to describe the poorer classes under treatment in mental institutions was offensive both to the patients and to their relations. It was hoped that the Mental Health Act which was at the time going through Parliament would help to improve the whole situation. It aimed at making it possible to treat cases of insanity without having to certify them. It was hoped that in this way cases could be treated in general hospitals and hot have to be admitted to mental hospitals at all.

From this time the general attitude towards mental illness improved, though the change was gradual. In 1931 patients could as last be admitted on a voluntary basis rather than always being certified. That was a great advance and progress has continued up to the present time when a great many cases are cared for within the community outside the hospital.

There is also a great improvement in the treatment of children. No longer are the retarded cruelly labelled idiots. Children are carefully assessed as to their abilities with the aim of helping them to reach their maximum potential. Naturally this does not always happen any more than it does in the mentally normal person.

Treatment is not only well understood but also well organised. Soon after the Second World War, out-patient departments were opened to deal with various categories of patient. A special provision was made for epileptics in the community and an occupational centre for defectives was started. There were clinics for delinquents and it was decided to have a child guidance clinic and a hostel for maladjusted children.

Within a year the hostel was opened. It was housed in a former curates' hostel called "Littleford" and sixteen children from five to sixteen years of age lived there. There was a school in the hostel for those who needed it but most of the children were able to attend local schools and return to the hostel for treatment afterwards. The results were good and they rarely had to stay for more than eight months, by which time they were able to return home.

Five years later "Littleford" was required by its former owners so another house was bought to replace it. It was renovated and was known as "Kempton" where the same form of treatment was continued.

Children who needed residential care were looked after in a bungalow in the hospital grounds.

From the start, good use was made of the grounds and these have been added to over the years. In 1911 a further twenty-eight acres were bought and some were used to build a dairy. The land cost £9,876 an interesting comparison with the original cost of the seventy-five acres bought for £14,000 in 1876.

At this time, two padded rooms were built, one for the women and one for the men. As treatment progressed, they were no longer needed

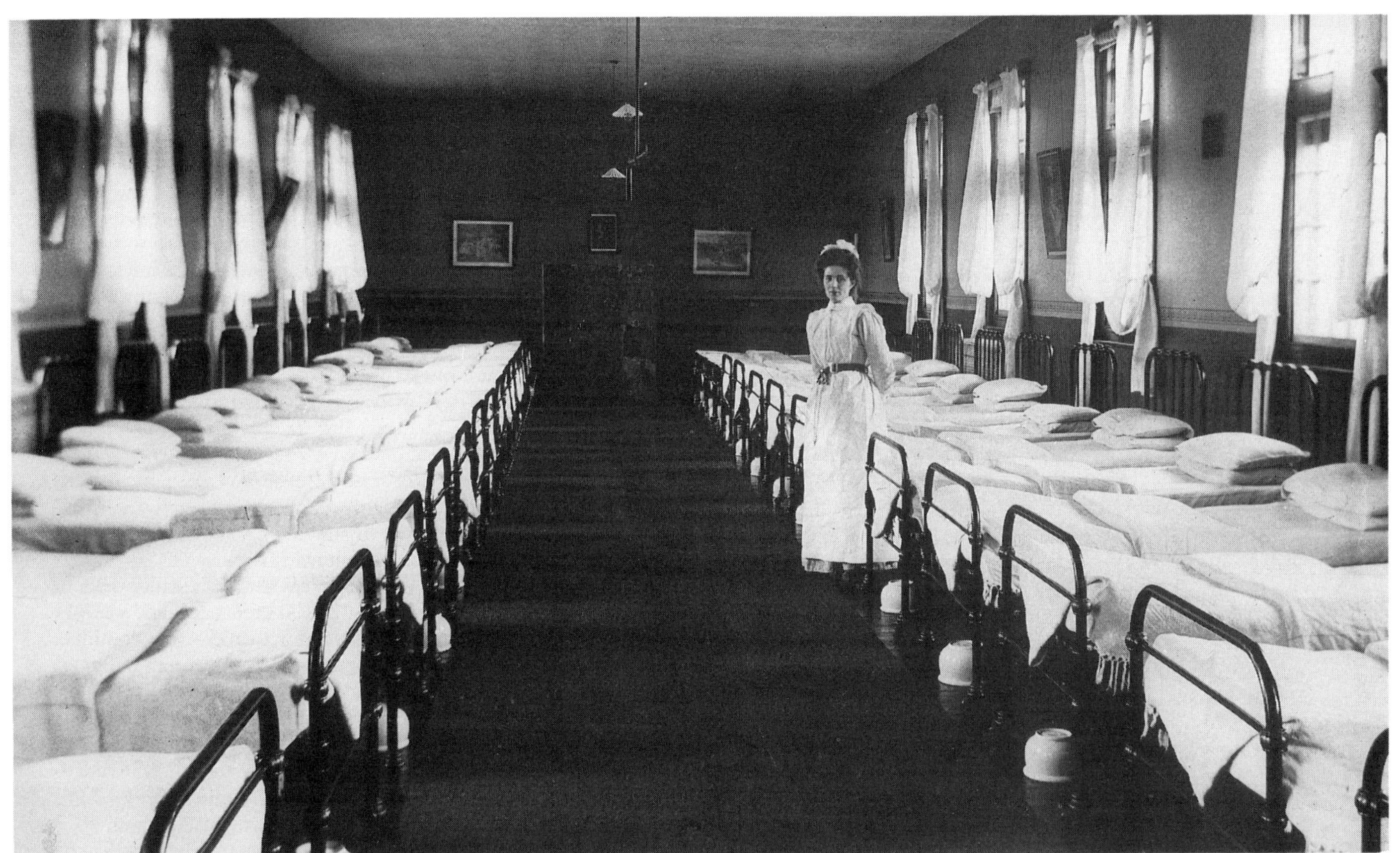

The very overcrowded wards.

but it was not until 1961 they were finally removed. Also, the larger rooms had been divided by glass partitions and these were removed at the same time.

Gradually the patients were becoming less restricted and in 1964 the corridors between the male and female sides were opened from noon till eight o'clock allowing patients to join togther for meals and recreation. Long before that time, more freedom was encouraged, in the first place by having some unlocked wards and villas so the patients were free to walk in the grounds. Some who were able to do so went shopping in the town unaccompanied. It was all pointing to the direction of the present attitude advocating complete freedom with a minimum of supportive care.

By the 1950s the hospital was becoming more and more like a complete community. By the end of the decade there was a professional hairdresser with salons for both men and women.

When the eight foot walls round the exercise yards were demlished in 1960 the bricks were salvaged and used three years later to build a cricket pavilion. The small panes of glass which were used in the hospital windows were replaced by large panes; there was no longer the constant risk of excitable patients smashing them. Treatment was still advancing, and at last overcrowding which had made nursing so difficult, was improving.

At one time things were so bad, it must have taken a very devoted band of nurses to work in such conditions. The patients had to retire to their beds immediately after their meal in the evening because of their numbers.

The tables were cleared and all knives and forks checked and counted. The patients lined up behind their places at the table and removed their socks and shoes. When they had removed all their outer clothing and placed it neatly on the top of the table they went up the stone staircase to the ward. The beds were so close together they had to get into them from the foot.

The nurses at that time were responsible for the complete care of the patients, supervising the cleaning of the wards and the preparation to some extent of the meals. Large loaves weighing seven pounds were cut up with a device similar to a bacon slicer outside the ward. At the start of the hospital's history the bread was sliced at table using an ordinary knife. This once proved too much for a suicidal patient who grabbed the knife and killed herself. From then on, bread was never sliced in the dining room or ward.

Now it seems impossible such conditions could have existed. During the 1950s, a dental surgeon began attending twice a week, and ophthalmologist weekly and the ear and nose and throat surgeon whenever needed. A Derby and Joan Club started and it still continues to meet. Also the League of Friends was formed. Nine years later the members opened a patients coffee lounge. In 1975 the Womens Institute came to St James'. Meetings are still held in the hospital although many of the members now live in houses in the city. Also in the fifties, the new operating theatre was opened.

The committee continued to make its regular inspections and often found ways of improving the general welfare of the patients. On the matter of dress the aim had always been to get away from the institutional appearance. Whenever possible it was hoped the patients could have their own clothes but with over a thousand inmates it was not easy to ensure this was done. To make things easier and to get them to take a greater pride in their appearance, each patient was supplied with a coat hanger. This sounds trivial but it made a great difference and showed both imagination and an insight into the needs of a mentally sick person. The committee often saw ways of helping which would have been missed by less dedicated visitors. Over many years a dry cleaning unit in the laundry had been needed, by the end of the fifties it was installed.

Wards were changing from being numbered to being named. M1 became Beaton Ward after a former medical superintendent. To short stay patients it does not matter if the ward had a name or a number. In fact a number can make finding the way in a large rambling building easier for visitors. But people who have lived in an institution most of their lives look on it as their home. And the more things to remove the feeling of regimentaion the better.

There was a well known patient who helped to improve both his own and other patients surroundings. Edward King was a very fine artist whose works have often been shown in the city. When he first came to the city he was a prolific painter but when he was admitted to the hospital he lost all inclination to paint. With the encouragement of the staff he started to take an interest again. Fortunately his old skills were only dormant and he soon started to produce some lovely pictures.

Edward King painted a great many works showing the result of the bombing in the last war. In this way he has provided a lasting record of that time. There was no sign of lack of concentration. Whatever his problem was it did not impede his considerable talent. His paintings are beautifully executed with fresh lively colours. They hung for a long time in the hospital and now can often be seen in the Portsmouth City Museum.

From 1960-66, further improvements were made. Apart from the Nelson Ward, the Solent Complex was opened. It consisted of two admission wards containing forty beds and a day-hospital all being connected by a covered way. Also the Alpha Unit was started for the rehabilitation of drug addicts. By this time the area from which patients were admitted had extended to Petersfield, taking in a population of 375,000.

In the seventies, a bank opened a branch for the use of the patients, so staff no longer had to be responsible for the care of patients money. The safe keeping of valuables and advice on both legal and financial problems added to the overall value of the new arrangement. The service made life much easier for both patients and staff and was especially helpful for those who were about to return to the city after being in a sheltered environment for some time.

The Havant Day Hospital was opened in Havant to give the people of that area out-patient care. At about the same time the Alpha Unit was moved out into the city and M4 ward was turned into a day unit for Psyco-Geriatric patients. By now Nelson ward was a unit for treatment of alcoholics. Conditions were constantly changing as the needs of the population changed.

Another phase of the hospital was complete. This included the Milton Ford School where twenty-five children from ages five to fifteen recieved treatment combined with various types of education. There were also facilities for parents to attend with their children.

Now the hospital has passed it's centenary its almost impossible to visualise it as it was so many years ago, so many changes have taken place. But in one way it has turned full circle. The hospital opened with just over four hundred beds; for many decades there were over a thousand but now it's back to around four hundred again. There are many more patients than that being cared for but they are out in the city being looked after by the social services.

Though the hospital as far as numbers are concerned is back where it started, in every other way it is different. It is a far cry from the days when words like pauper patients and idiot boy were accepted as normal; when the staff had little and at one time no training; and what little treatment there was consisted mainly of restraint so that patients didn't harm themselves and those around them — this coupled with as much activity within the hospital and the grounds as could be arranged. A walk in the exercise area wet or fine was the aim.

Fortunately the diet does not compare though at that time it was carefully thought out to get the best results out of the food. It was still hardly inspired. A typical day's diet in 1880 consisted of:

Breakfast: 8ozs bread. ½oz butter. 1 pint of tea.
Dinner: 5oz meat. 1lb vegetables. 5oz bread. ½1 pint of tea.
Tea: 8oz bread. 2oz cheese.

Sometimes tea consisted of ½oz bread and ½pt ale.

The items varied from day to day and between men and women; the outdoor workers had a slightly better diet than those who stayed

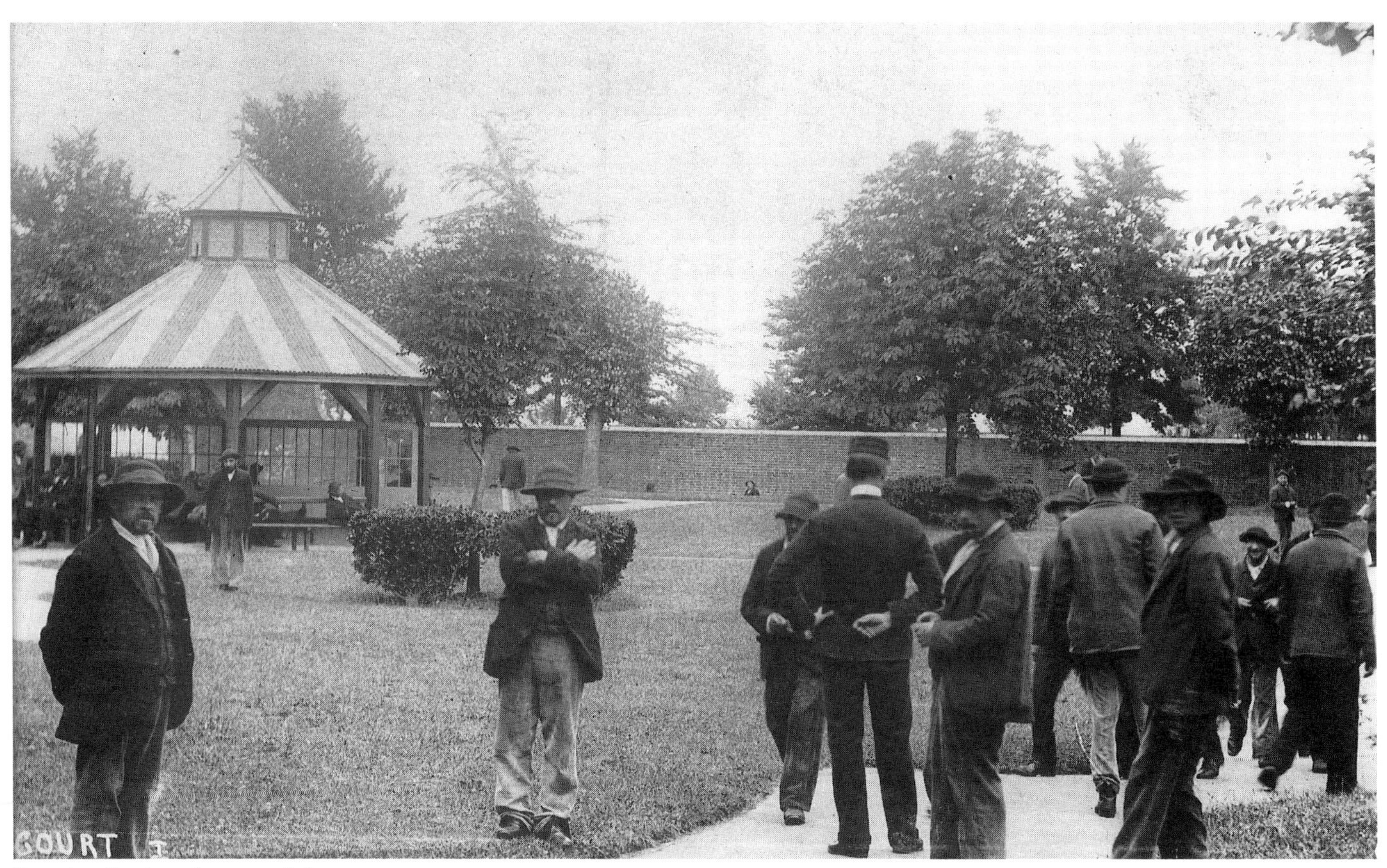

Exercise Yard at the turn of the century.

on the wards. Later, ale was removed from the list in the interest of economy. Though this diet would not be tolerated today, it was not as monotonous as it as first seems. The bread was baked in various flavours and I am sure was quite the best produced at that or any time since. During the war it was baked in brick ovens. When the Royal staff worked at St James', it was the high spot of the day when a piece of bread and dripping could be scrounged. It had a taste all of its own and has never been forgotten. Eating on duty was not allowed but in this instance it was done whenever possible and considered well worth the risk. It was really marvellous stuff.

Sadly, like the farms, the bakery is now closed. The original aim of making the hospital a self supporting unit no longer applied.

For several years St Mary's and St James' held joint clinics where consultants from both hospitals pooled their knowledge and ideas. These clinics were held at St Mary's and the patients from the assessment wards were often sent to St James' when they needed specialised treatment. From 1973 St James' became absorbed into the Portsmouth Group Hospital Management Committee and then both hospitals were administered from St Mary's. Therefore, after nearly a century St James' lost its independance.

The hospital which is now responsible for the joint management was the next to open. It was originally two distinct hospitals. The east wing was the Infectious Diseases Hospital founded in 1882. The west wing was originally the workhouse infirmary. The workhouse goes much further back, even before the Royal, as it was founded in 1845. The workhouse infirmary was added in 1860. So St Mary's General Hospital has in a sense two dates on which it could be said to have been founded.

Nearly ten years before the Infectious Diseases Hospital was opened, Dr George Turner became the first medical officer of health in Portsmouth under the Public Health Act. As medical officer he was greatly concerned about the lack of sanitation in the borough. The first thing he did was to seek Parliamentary sanction for the compulsory

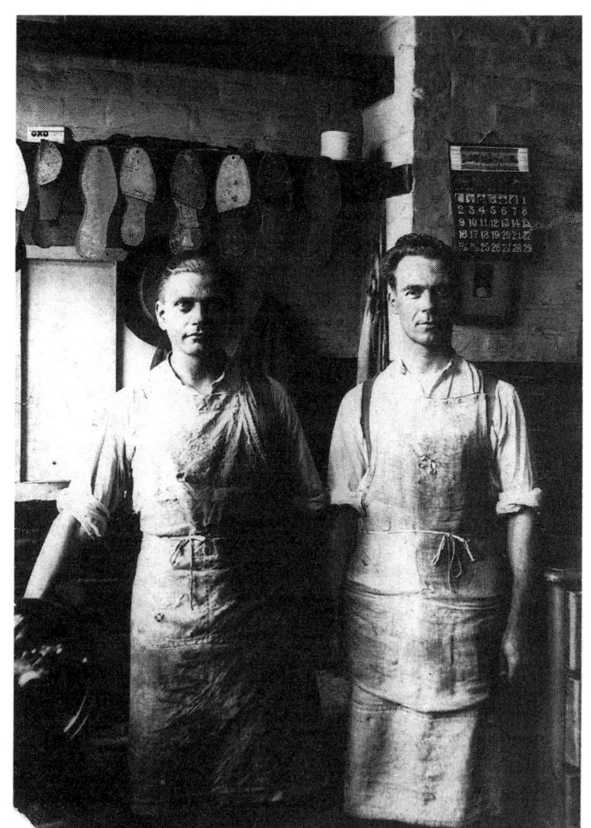

Two tutor boot repairers in charge of the repair shop, 1931.

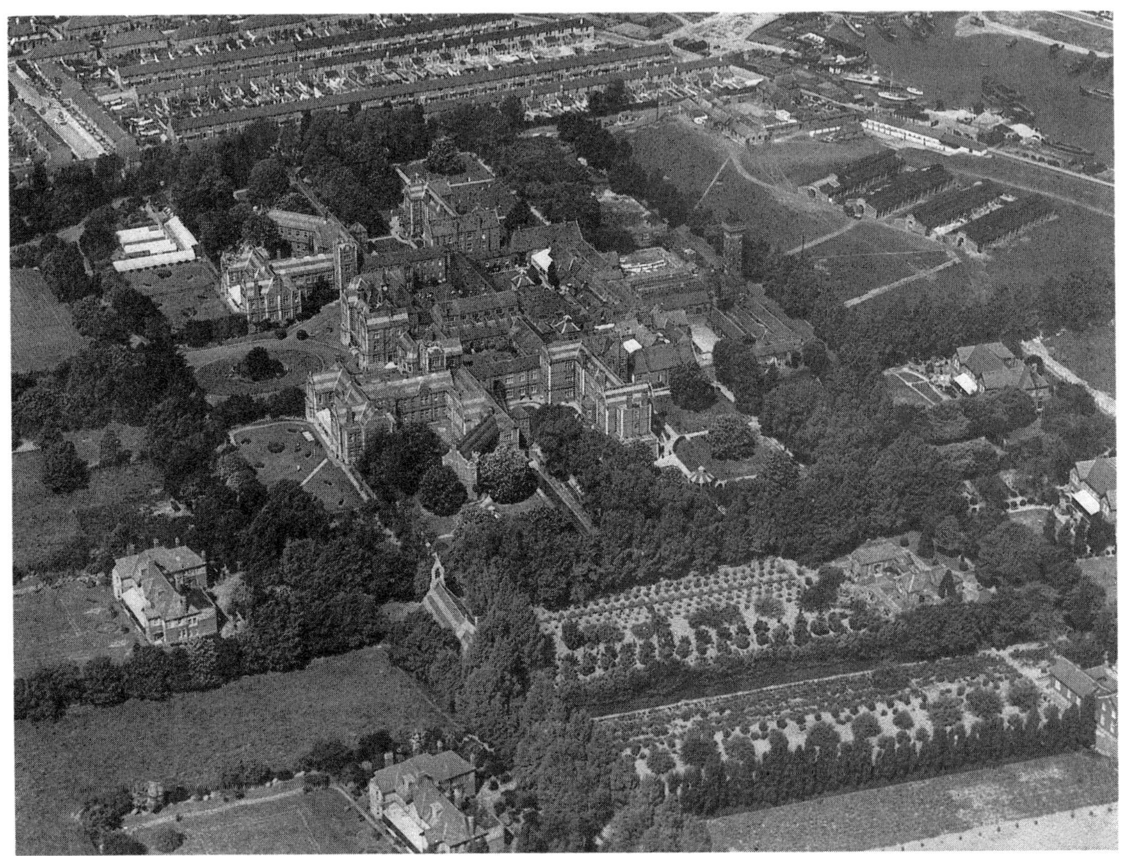

Overall view. 1933.

notification of infectious disease. The town council was not convinced that the trouble would be worth the results, but by 1886 they had to admit that the threat of an epidemic reduced its impact considerably. In any case he only anticipated an Act of Parliament which made notification compulsory.

He was very anxious to improve the general condition of the streets. Of the 19,000 houses only one third were connected to the main sewer and the sewer was far from satisfactory. There were four hundred and fifty manholes which released sewer gas. Although this was supposed to be deodorised with charcoal the people who lived near by complained bitterly.

As foul air seemed to be usual at that time these manholes must have been extremely noxious. Many of the houses which were connected to the unventilated cess pits had sewer gas in the houses and often several inches of contaminated water both in the yards and under the floor. The roads were full of holes which quickly filled up with water which had been thrown out into the street. Even the houses were not immune. The mortar was often mixed by using the water from the streets, so contamination was actually built into the houses.

After tackling the uphill task of educating both the people and the authorities in elementary hygene, Dr Turner went even further.

He started as an experiment a small isolation hospital. He bought a cottage in what was then the country and admitted two cases, one of small pox and one of scarlet fever. Both of these conditions had a high mortality rate. The cottage stood where the present east wing of St Mary's was built.

As was so often the case with innovators, Dr Turner was not appreciated by the people he was trying to help. When he became dissatisfied with the conditions in which he was expected to work, nothing was done. So he decided to leave the borough and Portsmouth lost a valuable and far seeing member of staff.

He went to Africa where he later concentrated on research into the treatment of leprosy. On reaching retirement age he returned to England and continued his work. It was then he discovered he had contracted the disease himself. Two years before he died in 1915. His name appeared in the New Years Honours List.

One of the great killer diseases was scarlet fever. When the first experimental hospital was opened, four hundred and eighty-three persons had in Portsmouth died that year. The classification of diseases at that time was interesting. According to a medical officer's report, although measles, small-pox, diptheria and scarlet fever were listed as infectious, tuberculosis came under the heading of constitutional. Typhoid did not seem to be taken as seriously as it is today. Because of years of soil contamination, it was endemic so perhaps the population had acquired some sort of immunity. By all accounts, recovery often took place in a relatively short time; few cases seem to have been admitted to the wards.

The foundation stone of the permanent hospital for infectious diseases was laid by the Mayor of Portsmouth, Alderman Whitcombe in 1882. Plans were drawn up by local builder Mr Tull and the buildings were completed and ready to be opened in 1883. They consisted of an administration block, kitchen and two pavilions for the accommodation of twenty four patients.

At the same time, the workhouse opposite continued to expand. A school had been built in 1863 and now in 1883 two imbecile wards were opened. So in a way the two hospitals were progressing together.

Like St James's the Infectious Diseases Hospital was under the administration of the health and housing committee of the town council. The committee consisted of representatives from each municipal ward in the borough together with the Mayor and three aldermen. St Mary's however came under the authority of the board of guardians. In 1898 the infirmary was built near the workhouse and Dr Charles Knott was appointed medical superintendent. Although his stay was relatively short — he died in 1908 — the work he did was appreciated throughout the country. He was so dissatisfied with the nursing standards that he started a training school for nurses. The guardians were so impressed by the results that the idea was soon adopted by other boards of guardians. In this way Dr Knott's influence extended far beyond his own town. His work did not go unacknowledged for he recieved the honour of the Order of St John of Jerusalem.

The Infectious Diseases Hospital continued to enlarge. When the matron Miss A.M. Autram was appointed three years after the opening, a lodge was built. Soon afterwards a pharmacy, lecture room and further domestic offices were added. Miss Autram continued as matron for seventeen years during which time rapid changes took place. By 1922 the hospital had been enlarged on six occasions. By that date there were eleven pavilions with two hundred and sixty five beds in all. One of the blocks was unusual for that time. It consisted of four wings radiating from a central room. Each wing was made up of five single-bedded rooms each room separated from the next by a glass partition. From the central room the nurse had a perfect view of all twenty patients whilst they were effectively isolated from each other. At that time the average annual intake of patients was over one thousand.

There were also thirty-two beds for advanced cases of tuberculosis. These patients were transferred to Langstone Sanatorium when their condition improved sufficiently, or when they no longer needed the specialised treatment only available at the Infectious Diseases Hospital. The nearness of the Infectious Diseases Hospitals to St Mary's made it convenient for the patients to attend the latter's X-ray department for their regular check-ups during their stay. This regular journey across the road was a welcome break in the monotony of many months spent on the wards. New drugs and the introduction of mass radiography units at the end of the last war have done much to stamp out this disease. The mass radiography unit was based at St Mary's and was opened by the deputy chief medical officer of the Ministry of Health on July 27th 1944 with Mr Cecil Ashwin as superintendent radiographer and Dr McLachlan the medical officer in charge.

The unit stayed at St Mary's for part of the year and the rest of the time it toured in the district in a large mobile van. It was based sometimes in the car park in small towns and sometimes in the grounds of large factories. Many early cases were diagnosed; treatment was correspondingly short and by checking contacts, the infection was contained. Even with people working in a fairly close atmosphere, positive results were rare. The general improvement in living standards no doubt contributed to the vast reduction in the number of people suffering from the disease. It was at about this time that the sanatorium at the end of Locksway Road was no longer required.

During the thirties children would cross the road rather than pass the Infectious Diseases Hospital. It held a dreadful facination for them. The distinctive infectious disease ambulance had the same effect. Perhaps it was the fear of what they hoped would remain the unknown.

On July 14th 1938, a new extension was opened by Sir Arthur McNaily K.C.B. M.D. FRCP the Ministry of Health and Board of Education's chief medical officer. It consisted of a two-storey block, each floor containing two large wards and four side wards with sixty-four beds in all. There was also an isolation ward on the cubicle system with five childrens cubicles in each arm making twenty beds in all.

To complete the extension, the two nurses homes were enlarged so as to be able to accommodate ten sisters and thirty nurses. A sisters lodge and a new kitchen and dining-room were also added.

Next year saw the installation of an iron lung, a very necessary addition to any hospital where poliomyelitis patients were treated. There were many references to fund raising for the unit, especially when it became the polio. unit in 1953. One example was the presentation of a specially designed chair by the Fareham Round Table on January 15th 1959.

It is the small things which can hit the headlines as well as the vital ones. In 1957 it was decided that ale and stout would no longer be supplied by the Health Service. It was thought that the extra nourishment provided could be administered more cheaply by other means. It was an unpopular decision and considered to be penny pinching.

Although there was an active League of Friends at St Mary's, one had not yet been formed at the Infectious Diseases Hospital. In 1957 this was rectified and they were soon actively concerned with the welfare of the patients.

Three years later, on May 17th, the hospital's name was changed to Priorsdean. There was still a need for wards for patients with infectious diseases but because of various programmes of immunisation, the number of beds could be greatly reduced. The hospital was now dealing with a wide range of complaints. A renal unit was opened and by 1967 a unit for regular treatment by dialysis was added. The following year the name of the hospital was changed again when it was amalgamated with St Mary's. It became the east wing of St Mary's. Now occupying each side of Milton Road and is now a large general hospital.

St Mary's has always been the larger of the two hospitals. In 1927, when there were two hundred and sixty-seven beds in the Infectious Diseases Hospital, St Mary's Infirmary had eight hundred and nine. The grounds of the Infectious Diseases Hospital are fairly uniform but around St Mary's are enormous contrasts. Its distant roots are still there.

Facing St Mary's Road is the old St Mary's workhouse, an imposing building with a well proportioned facade. Over the door is carved the date 1845. Although it is now in a poor state of repair, it must have been a very fine building in its day. Near there are the old Portsea Union vagrant wards. Separated by a plaque are two doors, one marked Men and the other Women. The plaque is dated 1881 and has the name of the architect Alfred Bone and the builder David Lewis, as well as the names of the chairman John Sapp and the vice-chairman C.T. Cunningham. A very austere looking building it could in no way be described as welcoming, but it was in use for many years.

On the laundry is another stone bearing the date August, 1895. This stone was laid by the chairman of the board of guardians, Mr F.C. French. The builder was Henry Jones. There are several more names but they have become indistinct with age. Another stone which commemorated the purchase of twenty three and a half acres of land in 1890, was lost, but recovered years later outside an antique shop in 1968. Where it had been and how it got outside the shop is shrouded in mystery. At the time it was put into position, the wall along St Mary's was built.

In common with the Infectious Disease Hospital, additions to St Mary's continued. In 1908 another block was built consisting of four wards for T.B. patients. Four years later four more wards were added.

With St Mary's and the Infectious Diseases Hospital both increasing their building programmes, there must have been a hive of industry on both sides of Milton Road. Not only wards were built. The Infectious Disease Hospital had a steam laundry and a steam disinfectant unit for clothes and St Mary's had a new operating theatre. The bed complement was increased by four hundred and sixty two beds.

The jurisdiction of the guardians came to an end, the Public Assistance authority took over in 1930. They decided that ratepayers could be admitted for both medical and surgical treatment and considered that by this time, St Mary's was already a general hospital and not just a workhouse infirmary. A small fee would be charged according to means. In no case would it exceed a guinea a week. In this way it was thought the stigma of the poor law would be overcome.

Early in the history of the hospital, the recruiting of nurses naturally was one on the prime responsibilites of the matron and the committee. Reading the notes made by the selection board is interesting. It certainly was not all plain sailing. The previous employment of the applicants varied, and the reasons for failure were many. There were cashier's tailoresses, florists and lady's maids to name but a few. One described herself as divorced but did not even make the first interview. Another at 5ft was considered too short, though why she made the interview is surprising as her height must have been apparent when she filled in her form. Another was too young at nineteen, one had poor sight and another a rude and unpleasant manner.

No doubt many did get past the interview, but not all reached the end of their training. "Rather tactless with patients and undignified with juniors" was the downfall of one. "Not energetic and inclined to be an agitator" was considered to be the problem with another. "Very slow of comprehension — it's a wonder she ever managed to start in the first place." "Confessed to having broken open another nurses' money box" — a sure way of finishing a career — in nursing anyway. And for good measure one went off with a male attendant.

Some decided it was not for them. One poor girl had flat feet and after only one day, another decided it was all too trying. They were all thrown into a very different, unknown world so it was not surprising some failed. But many survived and had comments on their work such as — "A quiet, intelligent and capable worker," and "Very good nurse."

It all goes to show that even in the very early days of nursing the staff were carefully chosen.

The work was very demanding with long hours and few days off. How nurses survived the day with the uniforms of that time was little short of a miracle. Leg-of-mutton sleeves, tight belts and long unhygenic skirts sweeping the ground; high necklines and bows, or strings as they were called, under their chins. It is difficult to remember when strings for staff nurses were no longer a part of the uniform. They were still in use during the last war. But their passing couldn't be regretted; they added nothing to efficiency and a great deal to discomfort.

The Public Health Authority took over from the Public Assistance Authority three years later. There was yet another change when the National Health Service became the governing body in 1948.

Shortly after the guardians gave up control, new gates were built which made access much easier. There was now a clear entrance from Milton Road with room for ambulances and garages, there was also a flat for the drivers. At this time it was found that the X-ray department was no longer able to cope with the extra work load, and a new Unit was built which would be able to deal efficiently with the rapidly increasing size of the hospital. A Dental Department was next with two surgeries and a waiting room. All these additions meant more staff. Just before the Second World War, huts were put up as a

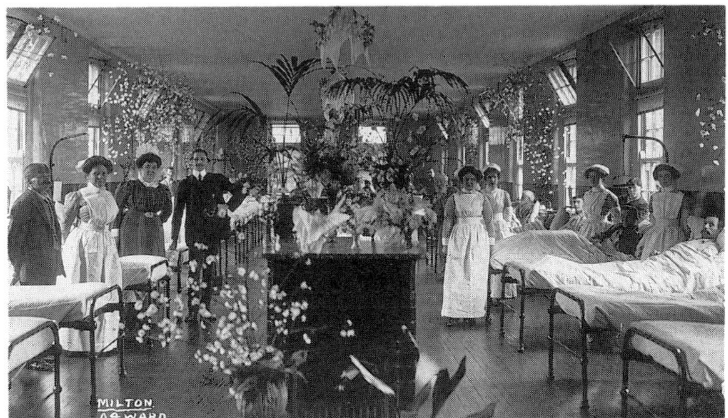

Ward St Mary's Hospital 1912.

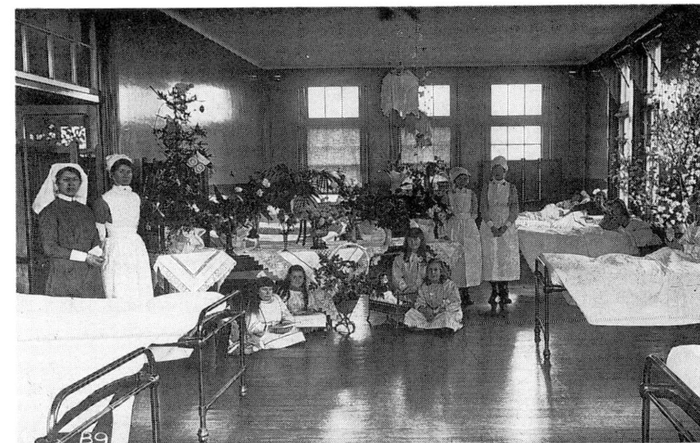

St Mary's Hospital Children's Ward 1922.

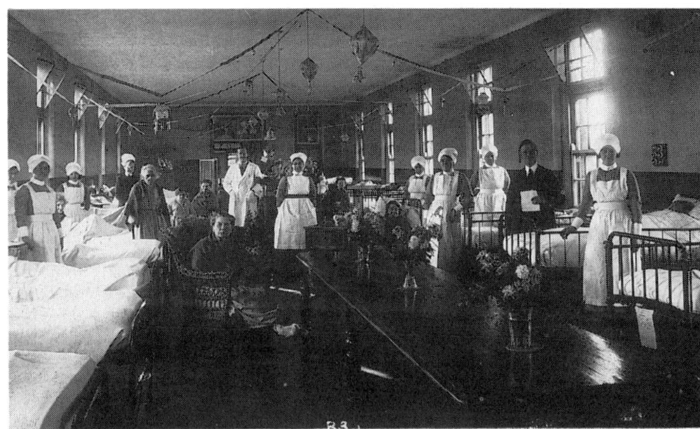
St Mary's Hospital Women's Ward.

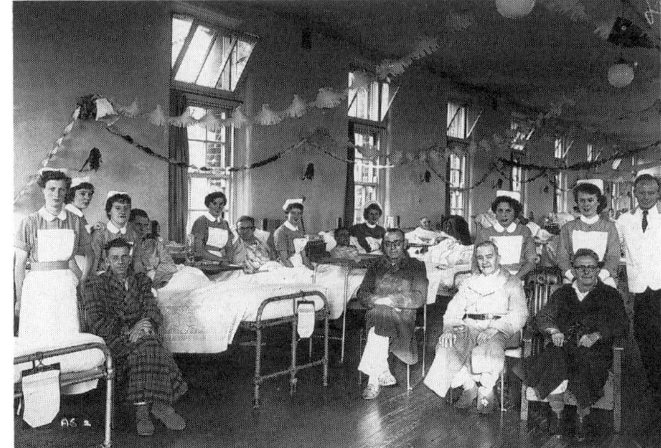
St Mary's Hospital Men's Ward 1945.

temporary measure for nurses' rooms.

Fortunately St Mary's was not bombed to the extent of being unable to carry on but the raids which did occur caused great inconvenience. There was extensive damage to the nurses' quarters, where eighty rooms were destroyed, together with the common room, the kitchen and matron's rooms. Troops were called in to help with the salvage work and the hospital managed to continue. Taking in patients from the Royal and the Eye and Ear must have added to the problems. Had hospitals not helped each other at that time the difficulties for the patients for the duration of the war would have been even greater.

After the war, fund raising for the polio unit continued. During that decade, the disease was still prevelant and being such a disabling condition, especially amongst young people, it naturally attracted much sympathy. In 1957 a polio respiratory unit was set up in the Infectious Diseases Hospital and shortly afterwards a central laboratory research unit was opened.

Now the disease is extremly rare because of the concentrated immunisation programme pursued over the years. From a national total of around four thousand a year in the days just after the war, the incidence has now been reduced to one or two cases. Immunisation has been reducing the severity and number of infectious conditions for a very long time.

In 1823 when the Portsmouth General Dispensary was being discussed, the establishment was described as being "for the purpose of supplying medicines and advice in accident and sickness — and the general encouragement of the Vaccine Inoculation is also the object of the establishment." This was at that time directed to the control of smallpox, of which there was an upsurge every ten years.

Neither smallpox nor polio are treated in Portsmouth now and there is just one ward in St Mary's east wing for the care of infectious diseases, which shows the enormous strides taken in the prevention of disease by various programmes of immunisation followed since the days of the Portsmouth Dispensary.

The past keeps reasserting itself in the history of the Portsmouth hospitals. In 1954 the Countess of Malmesbury presented the prizes at a ceremony at St Mary's Hospital. Nearly fifty years previously she had presided at the opening ceremony on the second day of the Great Trafalgar Exhibition in aid of the Royal.

Also in 1954, on June 19th, Miss Patricia Hornsby-Smith, parliamentary secretary to the minister of health opened the new wing operating theatre. The suite was made up of twin theatres which cost £1000 to equip and the building another £40,000.

It had been felt for a long time that St Mary's should have its own chapel. Funds were raised by the League of Friends, helped by the staff, patients, ex-patients, St Christopher's Hospital Fareham, and last but not least, the Reverend John Burt whose idea it was.

The foundation stone was laid by Lady Willis in July 1956, and the building was completed by October 18th 1959, the dedication being performed by the Reverend B.P. Robins, Assistant Bishop of Portsmouth.

There were protests after the ceremony because only an Anglican priest was present. Other denominations naturally felt they should have been represented. The Bishop of Portsmouth stepped in and assured those concerned that there had been a misunderstanding.

It was a pity that there should have been discord at the start of the chapel's life as it is a most interesting building with many dedications and whose furniture and furnishings show great ingenuity. An enormous amount of thought has gone into the making of this chapel.

St Christopher's Hospital presented the picture which hangs over the altar. It is a reproduction of Rubens "Descent from the Cross." The original which hangs in Antwerp Cathedral. Other parts of the building are the result of much investigation into antique shops, auctioneers rooms, and demolished buildings.

The carved oak panels of the altar-piece are seventeenth century and were found in a secondhand shop, possibly part of an old fire surround. The rest of the wood work was rescued by the chapel architect, Mr Ken Makins, from a seventeenth century shop front which was being demolished in Alverstoke. The oak panelling in the sanctuary, the wood for the altar, the bishops chair, the gallery and the screen at the back of the chapel all came from St Agatha's in Charlotte Street.

St Michael's Church, Southsea was being demolished at the time but the gates were saved and were used for the entrance to the hospital chapel. The sanctuary is lit by an antique Italian candelabra found in a Chichester saleroom.

A statue of the Virgin Mary was presented by friends in memory of Betty Wren, one time district midwife. There is also a memorial to all the nurses who died in the 1939/45 war. But not all the gifts are memorials. Some are there to give thanks for the recovery of relatives or friends who were treated in the hospital.

There was a rare event for the hospital chapel when one of the ward sisters was married there. Permission had to be granted by the Archbishop of Canterbury before the wedding could take place. On

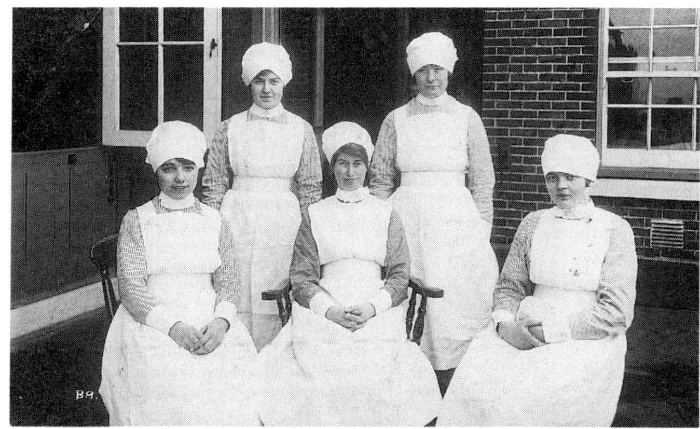

Pre war group. With all junior nurses observing the rule – "no hair to show beneath the cap."

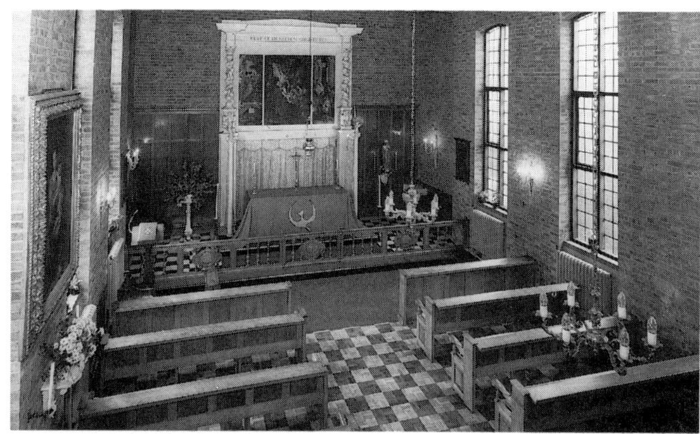

Interior of St Mary's Chapel.

August 6th 1979, the chapel was decorated with flowers and proved to be a lovely setting for the ceremony.

Shortly after the building of the chapel, the Lord Mayor's Fund was designated to be in aid of the purchase of two cobalt units for the radio-therapy unit. These were to be housed in a new enlarged department with a far more comprehensive range of treatments, there were also in-patient facilities.

During the war the radio-therapy department serving the Portsmouth district was attached to the X-ray department at the Royal. There were two radio-therapy and two diagnostic machines, all in the same department. They came under the authority of one sister though there was a staff nurse radiographer supervising the treatment side.

The main radio-therapy unit for Wessex was based at the Royal South Hants Hospital at Southampton. There were two boarding out hostels and wards for patients who were too ill to travel or who were being treated with radium. The area of intake stretched from the Somerset border to the Isle of Wight and the Channel Islands.

Just after the war, there was a radio-therapy department at St Mary's which was separated from the diagnostic side, but compared to the new unit it was not large.

In 1959 the new unit was opened by Sir Stamford Cade, a specialist known internationally in this field. By that time there was a school of radiography at St Mary's. During the war students were trained at the Royal but usually there were the hospital's own nurses with only very rarely a student from outside. Again, the nearest large school was at Southampton. Now there is a substantial and flourising school of radiography in the Portsmouth area.

Naturally it takes a great many people to staff such a large institution and during working hours, many of them never meet. The days have gone when everyone knew everybody else. But this isolation is countered by the activities of the social club which caters for most leisure activities. It was started after the war and has a very large enthusiastic membership. The theatrical group has had considerable success with the annual pantomime.

At the same time as administration offices were opened for the whole group in 1957, the private wing was built. The gradual enlargement continued and when during the next year the Public Health Authority removed the ambulances to their new quarters in Eastern Road, the garage flats were converted into accommodation for the married medical staff.

The upgrading of wards was speeded up and the balconies were redesigned and turned into day rooms. The hospital was quickly shaking off its workhouse infirmary image which clouded its early years.

The names of the wards are mostly taken from towns in and around the Portsmouth area, whilst the nurses homes have names either from royal houses or stately homes.

The east wing has Buckingham House as well as Osborne House, and Broadlands. The west wing has Clarence, Windsor and Balmoral House. There is one ward called Jersey but the others are Alton, Exton, Blendworth and Catherington.

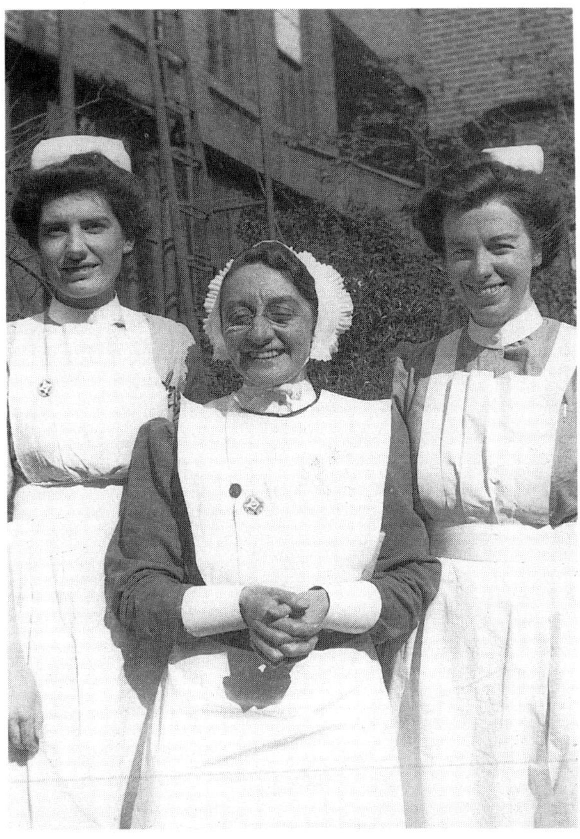

The Radio-therapy was mainly at the Royal Hospital. Sister Nottingham, with Nurse Morris and Staff Nurse Wardle. 1942.

The east wing goes a little further afield for names; Meon, Hambledon, Kingsclere, and Idsworth. The last one being the isolation ward.

The League of Friends always show great imagination with their projects. On July 19th 1979 they opened a suite of rooms so that relations of very ill patients could remain in the hospital overnight. It consisted of one double and one single room. There is also a kitchen and a rest room. Each bedroom is connected to the ward by telephone so that relatives of terminally ill patients can be called to their bedside at any time. It is a great source of comfort to feel it is possible to be with a loved one when their need is greatest.

The League also provided a creche for the children of staff who otherwise would be unable to work.

From 1960-70 a great deal of enlargement and reorganisation was going on. The telephone exchange was modernised so that calls for both St Mary's and St James' were routed through one switchboard. A new general practitioners maternity unit with twenty beds was built in the grounds. The intensive care coronary unit was opened and building work was started on a new two hundred bed maternity unit. This was subsequently opened by the Minister of Health.

There was a visit from Princess Margaret when she opened a new nurses home with bedrooms for sixty nurses.

On July 7th, 1977 another building was opened, which was very necessary to help care for the increasing number of geriatric patients in the area. This is the Amutlee Day Hospital, situated in the grounds at the back of the main hospital.

About the same time a unit for the care of cystic fibrosis was opened, a condition which has far more publicity now than it has had in the past. Therc had always been a large chest unit at St Mary's so the physiotherapy department has always been well equipped to deal with chest cases.

There is also a chest surgery department and these patients also need physiotherapy to ensure that they learn to breath correctly after their operation.

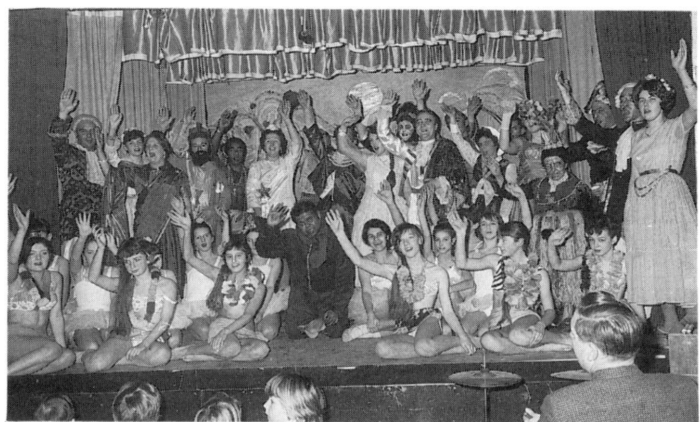

St Mary's Pantomime. As many as possible took part.

There is artifical limb centre so anyone in the area who needs this facility no longer has to travel to London or even further afield. It is a busy department because of the unfortunate increase in road accidents. Here again the physiotherapist has a big part to play by instilling confidence after a very traumatic experience.

The pathological laboratory which is in the east wing was opened by the Countess Mountbatten in 1950.

St Mary's has come a long way since the days of the Workhouse Infirmary. As one of the two general hospitals in the district it works with Queen Alexandra's hospital which has also made enormous strides since it was a military unit run by the Army Medical Corps. They both provide facilties for general medicine and surgery but complement each other in more specialised fields.

The particular specialities at St Mary's include gynaecological conditions, maternity and baby care. They have a well run premature baby unit of long standing. In 1968 for the first time a complete blood change was performed on a baby before birth. The name of St Mary's is synonymous with mother and baby care.

It is also known over a very wide area as an important centre for the treatment of renal disease in which great advances have been made. The same applies to radio-therapy, a highly specialised branch of medicine which is also based at St Mary's. Because of the very costly apparatus, these departments are usually some distance from each other which means some patients have to make long joúrneys to receive treatment.

Some of the clinics also serve specialist hospitals from other towns; Odstock Hospital, Salisbury for example.

So the hospitals work together. Queen Alexandra's is responsible for casualties, orthopaedics, eye, ear nose and throat and skin conditions, so the two city hospitals which were demolished are therefore resurrected within Q.A; The Royal's casualty and orthopedics, and the Eye and Ear's ear, nose and throat department.

Queen Alexandra is indeed a large hospital. There are eleven acres of flooring, one thousand and eight doors, and three-and-a-half miles of internal partitioning. There are also four miles of external beams. How many steps and stairs is anyone's guess!

But to go back to the start. As usual with hospitals it was not a particularly auspicious one! In 1853, just seven years after the foundation of the Royal, a military hospital was built near Lion Terrace. Previously there had been a barracks on the site. It was said to have been built with wood to house the troops during the war with the French, so it may well have been intended as a temporary structure. In demolishing the barracks to build a hospital, the events of 1690 were reversed. It was on that date the military hospital was replaced by a barracks.

The hospital remained until 1899 when the buildings were required by the admiralty. There was a fair sized military presence in the town so the hospital was still needed. To fill this need the admiralty made a provision for a new hospital to be built elsewhere. This became Queen Alexandra Hospital on the slopes of Portsdown Hill.

On December 13th 1900, a deed was drawn up between Queen

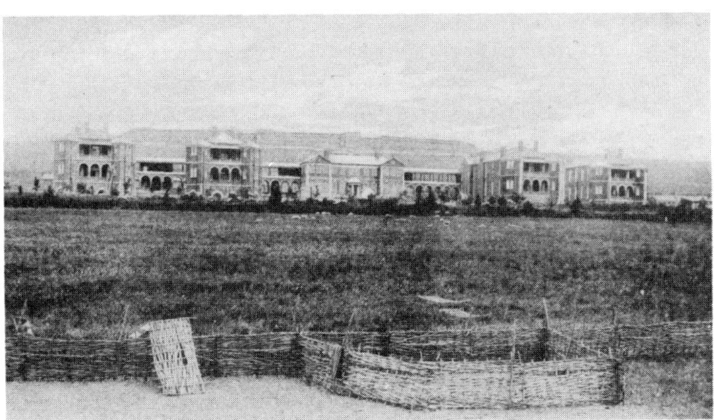

Alexandra Royal Military Hospital, Portsdown Hill

Victoria's Secretary of State for War and the Southwick Estate. It was to the effect that twenty-two acres of land at Wymering, the Wymering Farm Estate, would be handed over to the War Office.

The hospital was intended to serve a wide area. It would make provision to care for the military of the Portsmouth Garrison and for personnel from Weymouth, Dorchester, Winchester and Southampton. At first there were four blocks with accommodation for two hundred and twenty men. At first only one hundred men were admitted but this was soon increased to the planned complement.

Building was commenced in 1904 and the hospital was ready to receive patients in 1908. Lt. Col Bedford C.M.G. of the No 6 Army Medical Corps was in charge. Special ambulances were brought from Aldershot; there were two new motor ambulance wagons and as was usual at that time, several horse drawn ones. They were able to transport eleven patients at a time.

In each of the four blocks were two large wards of twenty-two beds and an officers ward with four beds. There was also a special mental ward with one padded room.

This hospital is still in use today but now it is virtually surrounded by the new and much larger institution. It is interesting to compare the two. It may well be one of the rare examples of the old style hospital working efficiently within the grounds of its far more modern counterpart.

Shortly after the hospital was opened it was found to be too small for its purpose. On the outbreak of the first world war, huts were put up in the grounds to provide a further two-hundred-and-eighty beds.

By 1926 acute cases were less numerous and the Ministry of Pensions took over the institution for the care of disabled service personnel from the Great War. It continued to fulfill this role until 1941 when the first civilian patients were admitted in January of that year. Some of these would have been cared for in the Royal had the facilties there not been limited by the bombing. Next year when the Royal wards were completely out of action because of two land mines which landed in the forecourt, even more patients were transferred to Queen Alexandra.

By this time both civilian and battle casualties were being admitted. With the D-Day wounded now coming into Portsmouth, the number of beds was once more inadequate. Building continued and the beds were increased to six-hundred-and-forty.

After the war patients both from the Royal and St Mary's continued to be transferred; orthopaedics from the Royal and geriatrics from St Mary's. The hospital was still caring for military patients but by 1951 all but one hundred beds had been taken over by the Ministry of Health.

When the hospital was first opened, a condition of its charter was that military patients would always be cared for. Although the patients now came under the Portsmouth Group Management Committee, military patients were cared for by Dr Preston, the unit's own medical superintendent. It was described at the time as — "a hospital within a hospital."

The hospital which was started as a replacement for the one in Lion Terrace was rapidly turning into a well equipped general hospital.

When in 1980 the new Queen Alexandra Hospital was opened there were still four beds reserved for war pensioners. Although it has far outgrown its original image, the agreement to have a place for these patients still holds.

When the new hospital was opended the old one was temporarily closed. All the wards have now been completely redecorated and they can take their place with the rest of the building. At the same time they retain their original character.

When the beds were taken over by the Ministry of Health in 1951, it was decided to make the hospital seem less like an institution by replacing the numbers on the wards with names. Numbers can still be seen on the side of some of the buildings but they have been removed from the wards themselves.

The first wards to be named were Edith Keen, Dickens, John Pounds, and Addison. Edith Keen was the matron of the Royal who was such a tower of strength during the war. At that time it was the women's surgical ward. Dickens was obviously after Portsmouth's famous son whose birthplace in Old Commercial Road is now a museum.

John Pounds was another remarkable man who was born in Portsea. He earned his living as a shoemaker when an accident in the dockyard forced him to give up working there. His disability did not prevent him earning a place in history. He was born in 1767 and his ideas in those days must have been revolutionary. He gave parcels of hot potatoes to the poor children of the neighbourhood and persuaded them to come to his workshop where he taught them the rudiments of learning. In starting the ragged schools he was well in advance of his time. There are two memorials to him in the city. The ward named after him and a plaque on the wall of a High Street chapel which reads — "He died suddenly on January 1st 1839 aged 75yrs. 'Thou shalt be blest, for they cannot recompense thee.' "

Addison Ward has had a name change now, but it was originally a tribute to Mr W.A. Addison, one time chairman of the Portsmouth Group Management Committee. Now it is Victory Ward in recognition of its adoption by H.M.S. Victory. It has a very nautical flavour with

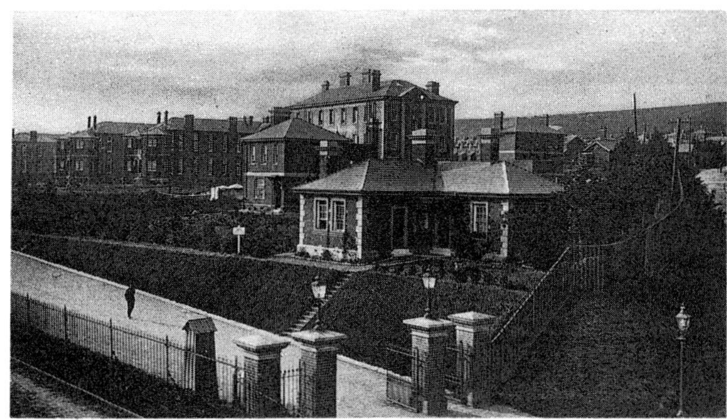

Hospital entrance from slope of bank.

the name over the entrance inscribed on a large blue and white arc. It is also a reminder of all the help given by the navy over the years.

Most of the names have obvious origins, such as Elizabeth Ward, and Diana Ward.

Off the main corridor are Mary, Anne, Philip and Charles. Also along there is a small X-ray department, all that remains of the original department.

Off the same side of that corridor is the Trevor Howell Day Hospital, opened in 1983 by Dr Trevor Howell F.R.C.S., founder of the British Geriatric Society. There is a plaque just inside the main door and a picture of the doctor in the main room of the hospital.

There are two entrances; one from the main corridor and one from the outside. This makes it easier for in-patients who have been in the wards for some time to attend as well as the out-patients who are still able to live in their own homes. The treatment available in the day hospitals is geared to prolonging the time elderly people are able to care for themselves.

Also in the old part of the hospital is the chapel. The plans for this had been considered in 1955 and the project started the following year, the chapel being finally dedicated on September 22nd, 1958. It had been hoped the stained glass windows saved from the Royal Hospital would be placed there but to date that has not happened. There is one coloured window, which is dedicated to the memory of William S. Chivers and Edith S. Chivers.

This was certainly not the first garden party to be held in the hospital grounds. The first took place just after the war in July 1946 and was opened by the Minister of Pensions. It must have been organised directly by the hospital staff, for the League of Friends, the usual power behind such functions, was not formed until 1952.

The friends held their first garden fete on June 12th, 1954 and they were carrying on a tradition which went back over a hundred years to the first days of the Royal. These fetes soon became an annual event and a prime source of funds for various projects.

In 1955 building began on a spastic unit and by December that year it was unofficially opened. The official opening ceremony was performed in June 1956 by Wilfred Pickles, a well known stage and radio personality of the time.

The League of Friends continued to work tirelessly and by 1962 had amassed the sum of £923. After further efforts, a new day room for patients was opened the same year. Seven years later they presented the hospital with a library. As usual they followed the pattern of other hospitals and concentrated on extra comforts which did not come within the state system.

From 1952 until 1978 they managed to raise £60,000. That meant a great deal of hard work and planning not only in raising money but in spending it wisely. The two group hospitals serve an enormous area. The Portsmouth South East Hampshire District includes the City of Portsmouth and its surrounds and serves a population of more than half a million. It is in fact the largest health district in the country.

When the new Queen Alexandra Hospital was opened by H.R.H. Princess Alexandra on June 25th 1980, she saw the result of twenty years of intensive work.

Because the building is sited on the side of Portsdown Hill, its construction is unique. Seven stories face south and there are only five visible on the north side. Consequently the entrance is on C level. The two lower levels are taken up by the engineers department, the staff dining room, the kitchen and stores.

The entrance hall would do credit to a first class hotel as would the kitchens which have a computer based system which speeds up the serving of over two thousand meals a day. It also gives warning should a patient order a meal which is inappropriate for any diet which may be part of his or her treatment. It was estimated when the new hospital was opened that apart from main meals, nearly one thousand people would be served in the coffee lounge each day.

In the main hall is a shop run by the League of Friends. Because of the size of the institution, a W.R.V.S. hostess is stationed near the entrance to take any patient or relatives to their destination should they be unable to manage on their own.

Naturally the main out-patients department and the more modern treatments, for example Hydro-therapy and the more specialised X-rays, are based in the new building. Should any of the patients in the old block need these treatments there are underground corridors connecting the old buildings with the new.

The Royal Hospital was for many years responsible for both casualty and emergency services. Now they are based at Queen Alexandra and take up a complete floor. The department takes in an area from Emsworth to Liphook, Gosport, Fareham and the whole of Portsea Island. In a full year there can be as many as fifty-five thousand patients, of which forty-eight thousand are first attendances. A tremendous amount of organisation must go into treating what works out to be one hundred and fifty cases a day, especially when it is realised that amongst this number are often very ill and badly injured people.

There are three one hundred and twenty bed units, one on each floor at levels D. E. and F. On G. level it is different. Here there are eighty-six beds for the treatment of ear nose and throat conditions in both children and adults. Here there are also facilities for mothers to stay

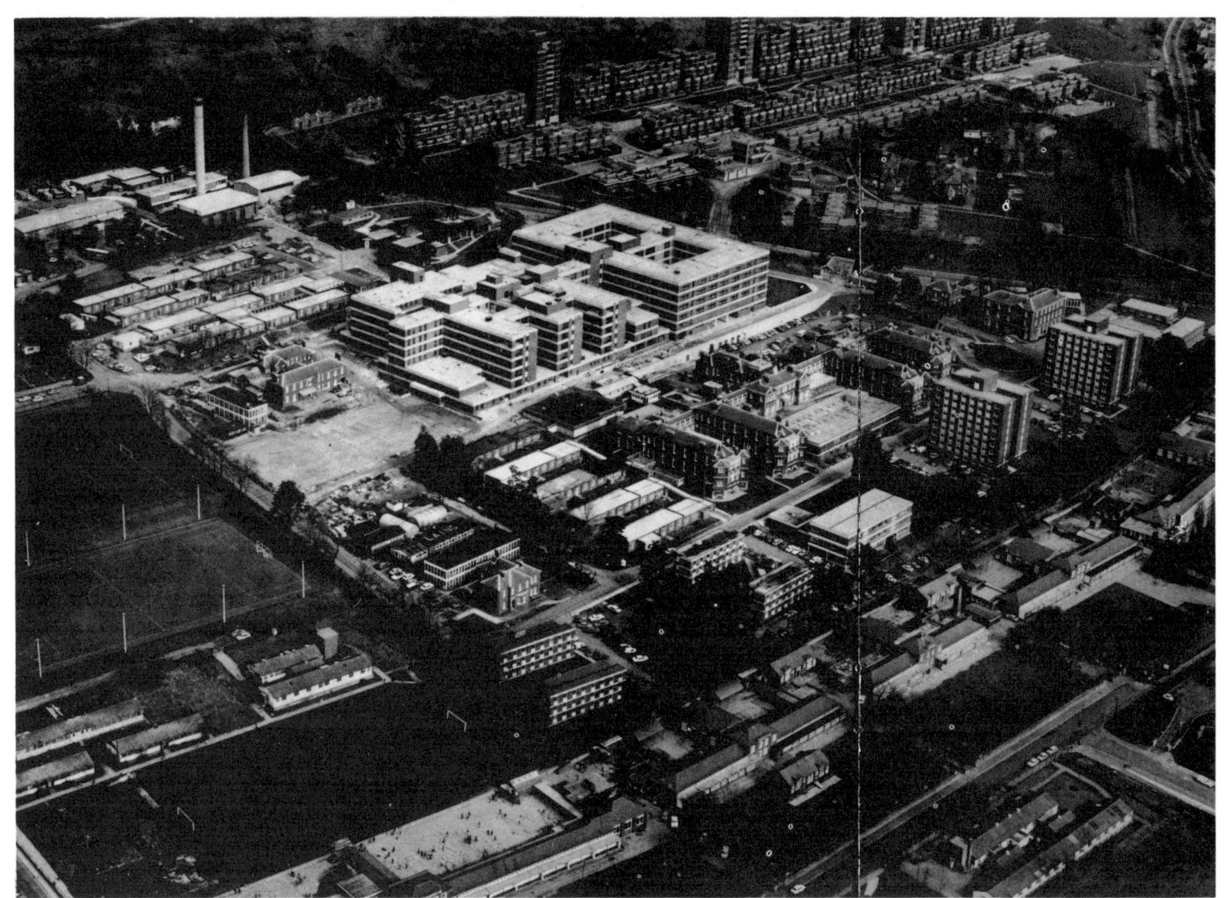

Queen Alexandra Hospital from the air.

in the hospital to be near to their children. Another part of this level houses the administraton offices.

When all the other departments are taken into consideration, general maintenance, clerical, domestic as well as doctors, nurses and auxillary medical staff, it is not surprising that when the new hospital was opened there was a staff of one thousand and eighty needed to run it.

Hospitals have come a long way since the Domus Dei, the Leper Hospital and pest houses for the victims of the plague. Here patients were simply isolated from their fellows until they died. There was a pest house near the dockyard on the edge of the common burial ground, a site chosen more for convenience than any consideration for the patients' feelings. The field was somewhere in the area between Unicorn Road and Fitzherbert Street. The dead were put into a shallow grave for the crows and ravens to scavenge. As in 1666 it was estimated that fifteen were being buried each day the whole area must have been frightful.

Even when the possibility of more scientific methods was realised, there were still gaps in performance as an inquest on a patient from the Grant Ward of the Royal Hospital showed. This strange affair took place in the late nineteenth century. The patient died as the result of a haemorrhage which the house doctor said had been caused by a chest infection. It was only when the nurse saw a blood stained razor on the bed that it was realised he had cut his throat. The coroner accepted the excuse that the error had occurred because, to quote the doctor's words — "He was a bearded gentleman." That this statement was accepted by the coroner without comment goes to underline the still primitive state of medicine at that time.

Though treatment and care have advanced considerably since that time, it is not so many decades ago that some of the methods were, to say the least, very unimaginative.

One young man can well remember his experience as a seven year old when he had his tonsils removed. It was just after the second war ended and the children were ready to go home on the day after their operation. He was singled out and told to open his mouth. The surgeon picked up a large instrument and quickly removed a small flap of tissue left behind. The child was then told to rinse his mouth. He recalled — "I remember it yet. It was a green liquid, It went down green and came up red."

Much earlier, just after the Great War another child had her tonsils removed but this time she went to a private nursing home. Here the treatment was more like the present day. Her mother was encouraged to be with her small daughter as much as possible and all her memories were pleasant. The operation was overshadowed by unusual attention; she was even asked what she would like for dinner, unheard of attention for young people in the early twenties.

For the most part, nursing homes today cater for the aged and those needing medical care. Between the wars it was different. One seventy year old lady remembers when as a ten year old she was bundled up in blankets and taken to a nursing home in the middle of the night. There she had an operation for an acute appendix; all this in the small hours of the morning. In those days the removal of an appendix was not the safe and simple procedure it is now.

Those homes were both staffed and equipped for twenty-four hour cover. Many elderly people can remember being nursed through major surgical and medical conditions in these establishments. There were also small privately run maternity homes in Portsmouth.

Now the emphasis is on longer and larger units, even the doctors' surgeries are joined together to form health centres. The only part of the Health Service which is getting smaller is in the field of the mentally sick or retarded and geriatrics. Here there is a firm belief in a more homely atmosphere, where a feeling of independence is fostered with a helping hand always available. It is interesting to see how opinions have changed.

Improvements in anaesthetics have made many surgical procedures possible. Transplants have become routine. But there are many people who still have faith in the simple remedies and herbal medicine has a place in present day treatment. It is impossible to guess what generations to come will inherit both in methods of preventing illness and health care. But it is fascinating to speculate.